Mental Health Interventions for School Counselors

CHRISTOPHER SINK
Seattle Pacific University

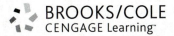
BROOKS/COLE
CENGAGE Learning™

Australia • Brazil • Japan • Korea • Mexico • Singapore • Spain • United Kingdom • United States

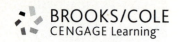
BROOKS/COLE
CENGAGE Learning™

Mental Health Interventions for School Counselors, First edition by Christopher Sink

Publisher/Executive Editor: Linda Schreiber

Acquisitions Editor: Seth Dobrin

Editorial Assistant: Rachel McDonald

Technology Project Manager: Dennis Fitzgerald

Production Manager: Matt Ballantyne

Manufacturing Buyer: Linda Hsu

Manufacturing Manager: Marcia Locke

Marketing Manager: Trent Whatcott

Marketing Assistant: Darlene Macanan

Marketing Communications Manager: Tami Strang

Art Director: Caryl Gorska

Permission Acquisition Manager – Image: Leitha Etheridge-Sims

Rights Acquisition Account Manager – Text: Roberta Broyer

Content Project Management: Pre-PressPMG

Production Service: Pre-PressPMG

Cover Designer: Lisa Buckley

Cover Image: Compositor: Pre-PressPMG

For product information and technology assistance, contact us at **Cengage Learning Customer Sales Support, 1-800-354-9706**

For permission to use material from this text or product, submit all requests online at **cengage.com/permissions**
Further permissions questions can be emailed to **permissionrequest@cengage.com**

Library of Congress Control Number: 2009940480

ISBN-13: 978-0-618-75458-8

ISBN-10: 0-618-75458-X

Brooks/Cole
20 Davis Drive
Belmont, CA 94002-3098
USA

Cengage Learning is a leading provider of customized learning solutions with office locations around the globe, including Singapore, the United Kingdom, Australia, Mexico, Brazil, and Japan. Locate your local office at **www.cengage.com/international**.

Cengage Learning products are represented in Canada by Nelson Education, Ltd.

To learn more about Brooks/Cole, visit **www.cengage.com/brookscole.**

Purchase any of our products at your local college store or at our preferred online store **www.CengageBrain.com**

Printed in the United States of America
1 2 3 4 5 6 7 14 13 12 11 10

Brief Table of Contents

TABLE OF CONTENTS   v

FOREWORD   x

Chapter 1: Attention Deficit Hyperactivity Disorder   1
Linda Webb (Florida Atlantic University)

Chapter 2: Externalizing Behavior Disorders: Supporting Students with Aggression and Violent Tendencies   16
Kerry B. Bernes (University of Lethbridge, Alberta, Canada), Jennifer I. Bernes (Registered Psychologist) and Angela D. Bardick (Registered Psychologist)

Chapter 3: Internalizing Behavior Disorders: Supporting Students with Depression, Anxiety, and Self-injurious Behavior   35
Christopher A. Sink (Seattle Pacific University)

Chapter 4: Eating Disorders, Obesity, and Body Image Concerns: Prevention and Intervention   63
Angela D. Bardick (Registered Psychologist), Shelly Russell-Mayhew (University of Calgary), Kerry B. Bernes (University of Lethbridge) and Jennifer I. Bernes (Registered Psychologist)

Chapter 5: Substance Abuse: Implications for School Counseling Practice   87
Glenn W. Lambie (University of Central Florida)

Chapter 6: Child Sexual Abuse   106
Carolyn Stone (University of North Florida)

Chapter 7: Students with Severe Acting-Out Behavior: A Family Intervention Approach   123
Keith M. Davis (Appalachian State University)

Chapter 8: Suicide Issues   135
Jill Packman (University of Nevada, Reno) and Catey Barber (O'Brien Middle School, Reno, NV)

Chapter 9: Learning Disabilities   154
Glenn W. Lambie, Kara P. Ieva, Stacy Van Horn, Jonathan H. Ohrt, Sally Lewis, and B. Grant Hayes (University of Central Florida)

SHORT BIOGRAPHIES OF CONTRIBUTORS   177
INDEX   182

Table of Contents

FOREWORD   x

Chapter 1: Attention Deficit Hyperactivity Disorder   1
Linda Webb (Florida Atlantic University)
Characteristics of ADHD   1
Recommendations for School Counseling Practice   4
Helping Teachers Acknowledge ADHD   5
Helping Teachers Become Aware of the Nature and Symptoms of ADHD   6
Anticipating the Needs of Students with ADHD and Planning Appropriate Interventions   7
Accommodating the Needs of Students with ADHD   7
Consulting with School Psychologists and Medical Professionals   8
Direct School Counselor Intervention   9
The Journey   10
Teaching Self-Monitoring Strategies   11
Working with High School Students   11
Stop and Think   12
Summary   12
References   13

Chapter 2: Externalizing Behavior Disorders: Supporting Students with Aggression and Violent Tendencies   16

Kerry B. Bernes (University of Lethbridge, Alberta, Canada), Jennifer I. Bernes (Registered Psychologist), and Angela D. Bardick (Registered Psychologist)

Characteristics of Externalizing Behaviors and Behavior Disorders   18

Prevalence and Etiology   19

Identifying Externalizing Behaviors   19

Assessing Externalizing Behaviors   20

Assessment Process   21

Recommendations for School Counseling Practice— Interventions   27

Behavior Management   29

Counseling Intervention   30

Educational/Vocational Planning   30

Summary   31

References   31

Chapter 3: Internalizing Behavior Disorders: Supporting Students with Depression, Anxiety, and Self-injurious Behavior   35

Christopher A. Sink (Seattle Pacific University)

Anxiety and Depression   36

Characteristics of Depression and Anxiety Disorders   38

Depression—Early Warning Signs   38

Anxiety—Early Warning Signs   39

From Early Warning Signs to Depression and Anxiety Disorders   39

Age of Onset and Prevalence Rates   40

Anxiety and Depression Disorders in Special Education Language   44

Recommendations for School Counseling Practice   45

Implement a Comprehensive School Counseling Program   45

Create and Implement a System of Positive Behavior Support (PBS)   45

Establish and Implement Prevention Activities in Conjunction with a School-Based Mental Health Screening Plan   46

Work Toward Prevention   47

Self-Injurious Behavior (SIB)   50

    Characteristics and Prevalence Rates   51

    Assisting Students At-Risk for and Engaging in SIB   52

Summary   54

References   56

Chapter 4: Eating Disorders, Obesity, and Body Image Concerns: Prevention and Intervention   63

Angela D. Bardick (Registered Psychologist), Shelly Russell-Mayhew (University of Calgary), Kerry B. Bernes (University of Lethbridge), and Jennifer I. Bernes (Registered Psychologist)

Overview and Characteristics of Eating Disorders   65

    Subtypes, Prevalence, and Long-Term Outcomes   66

    The BRIDGE Model of Healthy Versus Unhealthy Body Image   67

Recommendations for School Counseling Practice   69

    Eating Disorder Prevention in Schools   69

    School-Wide Prevention Programs   70

    Early Identification   74

    Early Assessment   74

Talking about Eating Disorders with At-Risk Students and Their Caregivers   76

    Making a Referral for Outside Intervention   77

    Supporting the Student in Recovery   77

    Phases of Intervention   78

Supportive Intervention Approaches for School Counselors   79

    Cognitive-Behavioral Therapy   80

    Guided Imagery   80

    Narrative Therapy   80

Summary   81

References   82

Chapter 5: Substance Abuse: Implications for School Counseling Practice   87

Glenn W. Lambie (University of Central Florida)

Characteristics and Warning Signs of Substance Abuse by Students and in Families   89

    Prevalence   90

    Potential Consequences   91

    Warning Signs and Identification   91

Children of Alcoholics   93

  Potential Consequences   93

  Warning Signs   94

Recommendations for School Counseling Practice   94

  Brief Family Systems Approach   97

  Motivational Counseling   98

Summary   101

References   102

Chapter 6: Child Sexual Abuse   106

Carolyn Stone (University of North Florida)

Defining Developmentally Normal Sexual Behavior
in Children   107

  Evaluating Children's Sexual Behaviors   107

  Level of Incidence of Sexual Issues   109

Signs of Sexual Abuse in Children   109

  Student Disclosure   110

  Interviewing Potential Victims of Child Sexual Abuse   111

Legal and Ethical Issues in Reporting Child Sexual Abuse   112

  Legal Responsibilities   113

  Ethical Issues   114

  Sexual Abuse in Schools   115

Prevention and Interventions   116

Summary   119

References   120

Chapter 7: Students with Severe Acting-Out Behavior: A Family Intervention Approach   123

Keith M. Davis (Appalachian State University)

Essential Characteristics of Acting-Out Behaviors   125

  Common Diagnostic Features and Associated Factors   125

Effective Family Interventions   126

  Specific Family Interventions   126

  Structural-Strategic Family Intervention   128

Resources for Professional School Counselors   131

Summary   133

References   133

Chapter 8: Suicide Issues 135

Jill Packman (University of Nevada, Reno) and Catey Barber (O'Brien Middle School, Reno, NV)

Background Information 137

  Prevalence 137

  Warning Signs and Characteristics of Suicide 138

Recommendations for School Counseling Practice 141

  Prevention 141

  Suicide Risk Assessment 143

  Interventions 146

  Postvention 147

Summary 148

References 149

Chapter 9: Learning Disabilities 154

Glenn W. Lambie, Kara P. Ieva, Stacy Van Horn, Jonathan H. Ohrt, Sally Lewis, and B. Grant Hayes (University of Central Florida)

Characteristics of Learning Disabilities 156

  Defining Learning Disabilities 156

  Prevalence 156

  Prognosis 157

  Observable Warning Signs—Internalizing and Externalizing Behaviors 157

Legal Issues and Legislation Governing Learning Disabilities 159

  Civil Rights Legislation 159

  Exceptional Education Legislation 162

  Diagnosing a Learning Disability under IDEIA (2004) 165

Recommendations for School Counseling Practice 167

  General Intervention Strategies 167

  Counseling Services 170

Summary 172

References 172

SHORT BIOGRAPHIES OF CONTRIBUTORS 177

INDEX 182

Foreword

Maintaining one's mental health can be a source of real worry. In an attempt to address this personal and societal issue, *Time* magazine's John Cloud (2009) overviewed the major disorders (e.g., ADHD, anxiety, depression, substance abuse) and how to "prevent" them. In a prophetic way, his remarks below provide an underlying rationale for this book:

> In any given year, appropriately 17% of Americans under 25 have a mental, emotional or behavioral disorder. (Over our lifetime, 46% of us will receive such a diagnosis.) If we reduce the proportion of young people who become mentally ill by even one-quarter, that would mean about 3.8 million saved each from what can turn into a lifelong struggle. (p. 76)

For children and youth with mental health issues to flourish during their school years and on into maturity, the contributors to this text and I believe that professional school counselors are able to be a key part of the solution. However, counselors must stay current and use relevant prevention and intervention strategies to be most effective. Along with leading school-based mental health researchers (Adelman & Taylor, 2009; Christener & Mennuti, 2009; Doll & Cummings, 2008; Taylor & Adelman, 2006), we promote here a collaborative approach to effectively address students' emotional and psychosocial challenges (Roberts & Mills, 2009).

Professional school counselors and other school educators should partner with mental health personnel, family members, and other community members to provide systemic prevention and intervention activities. Whether school counselors operate from a comprehensive school counseling program (e.g., American School Counselor Association's [2005] National Model) or not, competent responsive services (e.g., classroom or whole-school interventions, individual and group counseling) are essential to the welfare of students and their caregivers and families.

Turning best practice into real practice is a different matter. As most educators recognize, this collaborative aim is often elusive given the myriad issues schools, students, and their families confront each day. To further complicate the situation, the scope of students' psychosocial concerns appears to be growing (Center for Mental Health in Schools at UCLA, 2006, 2008). The enormous economic downturn of recent years, large school counselor caseloads (e.g., Lieberman, 2009; Rado, 2009), a lack of adequate time to do a job or run a comprehensive program (Dimmitt, Carey, & Hatch, 2007), as well as diminishing financial support for school- and community-based mental health services (see UCLA's Center for Mental in Schools, 2009; Whiston, 2004) intensify the need for readily accessible and quality resources to consult. In the climate that Cloud (2009) aptly describes, how do professional school counselors effectively address students' mental health-related issues? The American School Counselor Association (2009) devoted an entire issue of its *ASCA School Counselor* (volume 46, issue 5) magazine to an attempt to re-explore how mental health issues can be practically addressed in schools. Although the articles are helpful, they are, as one would expect from a magazine, only a starting point.

This book aims, therefore, to fill this gap in the practical school counseling literature by providing a reasonably concise, research-based, realistic "how to" reference guide for practicing K–12 and preservice school counselors (i.e., practicum students and interns). Chapters provide up-to-date information on the most common mental health or psychosocial/emotional issues and disorders facing schoolchildren and youth that can negatively impact their learning and long-term educational development. After providing an overview of each mental health concern, each chapter focuses on school- and research-based actions that are both prevention- and intervention-oriented. In other words, each contributor has made sure to include school counselor-educator actions that have demonstrated efficacy in school settings.

To ensure that the book resonates with both practicing school counselors and those in training, the primary authors of each chapter were specifically chosen according to the following criteria: Each one has served as a university-level school counselor-educator, worked with or in schools in a counseling-related capacity, and has published widely in the areas of their expertise. Furthermore, contributors have endeavored to write in a user-friendly way, translating, as much as possible, mental health vocabulary into educational concepts and language. We adopted the perspective that professional school counselors are educators first, not mental health therapists merely positioned in the schools. Plainly stated, wherever possible, we have attempted to minimize "therapeutic" jargon and emphasize what counselors could realistically do in a busy school setting.

The topics addressed in this book were generated by a thorough search of the education, counseling, psychotherapy, and mental health literature, and reviews from experts in the profession, as well as through many face-to-face discussions with practicing K–12 school counselors. The mental health issues or conditions most often cited as problem areas affecting student learning were attention deficit hyperactivity disorder (ADHD), externalizing behavior disorders (e.g., bullying, aggressive behavior), internalizing behavior disorders (e.g., depression and anxiety and self-injury), eating disorders, substance abuse, sexual abuse, family concerns, suicidal behavior, and learning disabilities. Readers will note that these topics are not exhaustive and they overlap, to some degree, in their etiologies and characteristics. For example, school counselors will observe what research continues to show that substance abuse often occurs in students with severe depression and students from troubled families (Office of Applied Studies, Substance Abuse and Mental Health Services Administration, 2007).

Each chapter has been organized in a purposeful way. To begin with, following introductory comments, each chapter presents at least one real-world case study of a student with a particular disorder. Second, the essential characteristics (e.g., age of onset, frequency of occurrence, key symptoms) of each mental health condition are addressed. Next, chapters include a "best practice" (intervention and prevention) section. Finally, each chapter provides a list of additional resources and references for the professional school counselor to draw on.

As a caveat, the chapters do not tackle in any depth the etiology of the condition discussed. The reason for this is fairly simple: this book is primarily concerned with giving school counselors useful preventions and interventions, rather than considering a variety of theories and equivocal research discussing the origins of each condition. The *Diagnostic and Statistical Manual of Mental Disorders IV–Text Revision* (American Psychiatric Association, 2000), for instance, provides no clear consensus on most mental disorders, indicating instead a mixed etiology. The same is true for attention deficit hyperactivity disorder and substance abuse, as well as other student conditions school counselors will deal with (e.g., conduct disorders, suicidal ideation, self-injurious behavior, etc.).

In summary, we feel that this book attends to a potential deficiency in the school counselor's prevention-intervention library. The text can be used to plan, implement, and evaluate school counselor/educational responses to students' mental health-related concerns. To be effective in these activities, however, K–12 school counselors need the latest information on these issues. Because the literature is growing so quickly that no one volume could ever fully consider the issues, continued reading of the most recent journals is a must. As general texts on school-based mental health, Doll and Cummings's (2008) and Christner and Mennuti's (2009) books are useful supplements.

Please let us know what you think about this volume and how the authors can improve each chapter for future editions. The editor of this volume can be contacted at his email address: csink@spu.edu.

★ ★ ★

The editor and contributors wish to thank Brooks/Cole Cengage Learning and its staff for making this book possible and shepherding it through the publication process. In addition, the editor expresses his deepest appreciation to Dr. Marianna Richardson at Seattle Pacific University for her many hours of preproduction editorial work. This text is dedicated to the professional school counselors who work selflessly each day to bring caring and healing to students and their families.

Christopher A. Sink, General Editior
Seattle Pacific University

REFERENCES

Adelman, H. S., & Taylor, L. (2003). Commentary: Advancing mental health science and practice through authentic collaboration. *School Psychology Review, 32,* 55–58.

Adelman, H. S., & Taylor, L. (2009). Ending the marginalization of mental in schools: A comprehensive approach. In R. W. Christner, & R. B. Mennuti (Eds.). *School-based mental health: A practitioner's guide to comparative practices* (pp. 25–54). New York: Routledge.

American Psychiatric Association. (2000). *Diagnostic and statistical manual of mental disorders IV–Text Revision.* Washington, DC: Author.

American School Counselor Association. (2005). *The ASCA national model: A framework for school counseling programs. Executive summary.* Retrieved September 9, 2007, from http://www.schoolcounselor.org/files/Natl%20Model%20Exec%20Summary_final.pdf

Center for Mental Health in Schools. (2006). *A Center policy report: The current status of mental health in schools: A policy and practice analysis.* Retrieved May 9, 2009, from http://smhp.psych.ucla.edu/pdfdocs/currentstatusmh/currentstatus.pdf

Center for Mental Health in Schools at UCLA. (2008). *Youngsters' mental health and psychosocial problems: What are the data?* Retrieved June 3, 2009, from http://smhp.psych.ucla.edu/pdfdocs/prevalence/youthMH.pdf

Christner, R. W., & Mennuti, R. B. (Eds.). (2009). *School-based mental health: A practitioner's guide to comparative practices.* New York: Routledge.

Cloud, J. (2009, June 22). Staying sane may be easier than you think. *Time, 173*(24), 72–78.

Dimmitt, C., Carey, J. C., & Hatch, T. (2007). *Evidence-based school counseling.* Thousand Oaks, CA: Corwin.

Doll, B., & Cummings, J. A. (2008). *Transforming school mental health services population-based approaches to promoting the competency and wellness of children.* Thousand Oaks, CA: Corwin.

Lieberman, B. (2009, May 18). *High school counselors brace for big caseloads.* Retrieved June 3, 2009, from http://www.theapple.com/news/articles/8424-high-school-counselors-brace-for-big-caseloads

Office of Applied Studies, Substance Abuse and Mental Health Services Administration. (2007, May). *Depression and the initiation of alcohol and other drug use among youths aged 12 to 17.* National Survey on Drug Use and Health (NSDUH) Report. Retrieved May 26, 2009, from http://oas.samhsa.gov/2k7/newUserDepression/newUserDepression.htm

Rado, D. (2009, May 27). *School counselors face big workload in Illinois: Trying to touch base with an average of 690 students.* Retrieved June 3, 2009, from http://www.chicagotribune.com/news/local/chicago/chi-counselors-west-zone-27-may27,0,3192041.story

Roberts, L. C., & Mills, C. (2009, May/June). Meeting students' needs. *ASCA School Counselor, 46,* 12, 12–17.

Taylor, L., & Adelman, H.S. (2006). Want to work with schools? What's involved in successful linkages? In C. Franklin, M. B. Harris, & P. Allen-Mears (Eds.), *School social work and mental health workers training and resource manual* (pp. 955–969). New York: Oxford University Press.

UCLA's Center for Mental in Schools. (2009). *National initiative: New directions for student support*. Retrieved June 3, 2009, from http://smhp.psych.ucla.edu/

Whiston, S. C. (2004). Counseling psychology and school counseling: Can a stronger partnership be forged? *The Counseling Psychologist, 32,* 270–277.

Chapter 1

Attention Deficit Hyperactivity Disorder

LINDA WEBB

Florida Atlantic University

Attention Deficit Hyperactivity Disorder (ADHD), one type of the several neurobehavioral impulse control disorders (Doll & Cummings, 2008), is one of the most frequently diagnosed disorders among school-age children (Barkley, 2006; Centers for Disease Control and Prevention [CDC], 2009). An estimated three to seven percent of the school-age population has ADHD, defined as persistent patterns of developmentally inappropriate inattention, hyperactivity, and/or impulsivity, with diagnoses of boys outnumbering diagnoses of girls about 2:1 (CDC). It is also important to note that for diagnosis some symptoms of ADHD must be present before the age of seven and create some impairment in two or more settings (e.g., at home, at school, with peers). In addition, there must be clear evidence of significant impairment from ADHD symptoms in at least one setting that is not caused by other psychical or mental disorders.

CHARACTERISTICS OF ADHD

As of 2006, 4.5 million children 5–17 years of age have been diagnosed with ADHD (CDC, 2009). The disorder's symptoms appear on average between 4 and 6 years of age, particularly the subtypes of ADHD associated with hyperactivity and impulsive behavior. The onset of ADHD for most children is frequently diagnosed when a child is in elementary school and problems related to

Caleb: A School-Based Case Study

Caleb is now 8 years old and beginning the second grade. First grade did not go well for Caleb. He was constantly reprimanded by his teacher for being out of his seat or rocking back and forth in his chair. When he was in his seat, he always seemed to find an object to play with in his desk. His teacher took "play things" away from him to redirect his attention. When he didn't have something to play with, he frequently interrupted the teacher and other students and had difficulty completing his work. Caleb's teacher and parents met and decided a daily note home regarding his behavior might be helpful. The teacher wrote the note at the end of each day. Most days the note was not positive. However, because he was successful in occasionally staying in his seat and completing his work, his teacher knew he was capable of on-task behavior and expected to see it more frequently. Caleb ended the year with average grades and his mother sat with him every afternoon, and sometimes evenings, to be sure he completed the work he had not finished during the school day. This was a trying time for both Caleb and his mother and many days there were tears. The summer went better for Caleb. He attended a day camp for eight weeks that provided a routine combination of outside and inside activities involving games, physical activities, and craft projects. While Caleb needed occasional reminders about taking turns and rarely attended to details when working on craft projects, he enjoyed the experience. He was well liked and considered "all boy" by camp counselors. Now the summer was over and Caleb was not looking forward to going back to school.

school performance surface (Shillingford, Lambie, & Walter, 2007; Zentall, 2006). Recent research has shown that disparities in the diagnosis of ADHD are a function of gender, race/ethnicity, language, and factors related to health care access and use (Visser, Lesesne, & Perou, 2007). While school counselors cannot use clinical criteria to make a diagnosis of ADHD (Harnett, Nelson, & Rinn, 2004), they can use those criteria to help parents and teachers think about whether ADHD might be a factor contributing to a student's behavioral concerns and/or underachievement and referral to appropriate medical and/or mental health professionals is required.

According to the most recent edition of the *Diagnostic and Statistical Manual of Mental Disorders, Text Revision* (DSM–IV–TR; American Psychiatric Association, 2000) and the CDC (2009), there are three subtypes of ADHD:

- *ADHD, Predominantly Inattentive Type* can be diagnosed if the criterion for inattention is met but the criterion for hyperactivity/impulsivity is not met for the past six months. Some signs of inattention include becoming easily distracted, making careless mistakes as a result of not paying attention to details, forgetting or losing items necessary to complete tasks (pencils, books, etc.), not following instructions carefully, or skipping around from one activity to another.

- *ADHD, Predominantly Hyperactive-Impulsive Type* can be diagnosed if the criterion for hyperactivity/impulsivity is met but the criterion for inattention is not met for the past six months. Some signs of hyperactivity/impulsivity include fidgeting or squirming when seated, running, climbing, or getting out of seat when quiet behavior is expected, blurting out, having trouble waiting turns, or being restless.

- *ADHD, Combined Type* can be diagnosed if the criteria for both inattention and hyperactivity/impulsivity are met for the past 6 months.

With an increasing emphasis on teaching young children to control impulses, pay attention, sit still, and finish tasks, it is not hard to understand why children with ADHD have difficulty in school. Struggles with independent seatwork, inconsistent school performance, poor study skills, low test performance, and disorganized desks and notebooks are common concerns (DuPaul & Stoner, 1994; Shillingford et al. 2007). Symptoms of ADHD related to inattention may not manifest themselves until middle or later childhood. The *No Child Left Behind Act* calls for Adequate Yearly Progress (AYP) for all students, which has some effect on students with diagnosed and undiagnosed ADHD.

Russell Barkley (2006), a prominent researcher in the field, has suggested that the major symptoms of ADHD are likely to vary depending on the specific situation of the student. For example, research suggests that those with ADHD behave better when participating in one-on-one situations, when doing tasks they find interesting, when being appropriately supervised, and when receiving frequent feedback for appropriate behavior. A student asked to complete independent seatwork in large classes, particularly with long or repetitive assignments, will likely manifest the symptoms of ADHD with predictable negative outcomes. Conversely, if this same student was seated near the teacher, given assignments that were shortened or chunked into smaller parts, and was provided with some immediate positive reinforcement for behaving appropriately, it is much more likely that student would be successful.

While Caleb, in our school-based case study, has not yet been diagnosed with ADHD, it is clear that his school behavior warrants a closer look. He is already losing motivation to come to school and will likely continue to fall farther behind in academic subjects if no accommodations or interventions are planned.

What are the likely outcomes if Caleb goes undiagnosed and/or untreated for ADHD? Caleb's level of symptoms may decline with age, but he will most likely continue to lag behind his non-ADHD peer group (Barkley, 2006). In other words, students with ADHD tend to not catch up to their age group in their capacity to inhibit unwanted behaviors, sustain attention, control distractibility, and regulate their activity level. Over time, untreated ADHD can lead to secondary behavioral and adjustment problems in part as a partial response to frequent and repeated failures (Barkley, 2006; Goldstein & Goldstein, 1998). Teachers and parents become increasingly concerned with the resulting under-achievement and social difficulties. Without assistance, Caleb may develop emotional problems such as anger, aggression, depression, or anxiety (Barkley, Fischer, Edelbrock, & Smallish, 1990; McKinney, Montague, & Hocutt, 1993), which are associated with Oppositional Defiant and Conduct Disorders (Biederman, Farone, & Lapey, 1992; CRC, 2009), creating more problematic behavior in schools. Other problems associated with untreated ADHD are lower academic grades and achievement test scores, and ultimately school failure (Shillingford et al. 2007).

What might we expect for Caleb if he is properly diagnosed and treated? While there is no cure for ADHD, there are medical and behavioral treatments that can help manage the symptoms and lead to more successful school behavior. Let's take a look forward to Caleb in high school, with successful interventions having been put into place throughout his school experience. As expected, Caleb's hyperactivity and inattention have improved as a result of developmental maturation. His physician, parents, and teachers have collaborated over the years regarding the appropriate use and monitoring of medication to help ease ADHD symptoms. At the same time, Caleb has learned more about ADHD as related to his school performance, as well as strategies he can use to reach personal and academic goals. By the time Caleb reached high school, he understood the importance of strategies such as sitting in the front of the class, using relevant technology, and finding a "study buddy" in each class to check assignments and important information. Caleb's mom still helps him "chunk" major assignments into smaller parts so he can mark his organizer with more frequent due dates leading to project deadlines. School personnel also wrote a 504 accommodation plan (U.S. Department of Education Office for Civil Rights, 2009) that allowed for lengthy exams to be given to Caleb in more than one sitting. While all students can benefit from these types of strategies, they are critical for students with ADHD. Caleb also joined the school's soccer team and provided positive energy and motivation to the entire team. All of this was not easy and took a collaborative effort involving Caleb and his parents, teachers, school counselor, and physician.

RECOMMENDATIONS FOR SCHOOL
COUNSELING PRACTICE

Teachers and parents or caregivers frequently look to the school counselor in cases such as Caleb's to begin determining the cause of behavior problems and academic underachievement. School counselors can provide information on ADHD to parents, caregivers and teachers, help develop educational accommodation plans for students who have been diagnosed with ADHD (by appropriate medical or mental health professionals), and provide direct service through individual or small group counseling.

When have school counselors had the opportunity to impact Caleb's outcome? Initially, the school counselor should become involved when the first consistent struggles were taking place. At that time, the counselor could take the opportunity to consult with Caleb's teacher, helping her to acknowledge the legitimacy of the disorder by providing information about ADHD. The school counselor might help teachers become aware of symptoms and interventions proven effective, and be involved in the intervention planning process. The following are school counselor interventions that can improve the chances of school success for students with ADHD.

Helping Teachers Acknowledge ADHD

While other disabilities are more clearly diagnosed and accepted, teachers generally have more difficulty accepting and accommodating students with ADHD. This may be due to the number of students who are inappropriately diagnosed, the inconsistency of the behavior of students with ADHD, or the negative media attention ADHD receives. Teachers frequently have difficulty accepting ADHD as a legitimate disorder due to the number of students labeled ADHD who have not received an appropriate evaluation and may actually be exhibiting primary symptoms of another disorder. This then becomes complicated by the fact that students with ADHD may "perform" in some situations but not others. This inconsistency is expected as a result of situational inconsistencies that improve or impair the chances that a student will be successful. The media also plays a role in the acceptance of ADHD as a legitimate disorder, and experts have felt the need to address this negative attention. A published International Consensus Statement on ADHD (Barkley et al., 2002) was based on research findings from a consortium of international scientists who are deeply concerned about the periodic inaccurate portrayals of ADHD in media reports and doubt the legitimate acknowledgement of the disorder among the public. A copy of the statement can be found at this Web site: http://www. russellbarkley.org/.

The frequent misdiagnosis of previous students, Caleb's own inconsistent behavior, and negative media attention to ADHD may have likely played a role in the teacher's hesitation to feel the need to accommodate Caleb. Caleb's teacher knew he was capable of on-task behavior because she had seen him succeed at it occasionally. However, the conditions under which Caleb was on task may have included a shorter assignment or high-interest assignment, more structured directions, or closer monitoring by the teacher. As many experts have noted (Barkley, 2006; Goldstein & Goldstein, 1998; Gordon, 1993), ADHD is not always about students knowing *what* to do, but about *doing* what they know. ADHD can become a disorder in which students have difficulty performing even if they know what is expected. It is important for school counselors to stay involved in these types of situations. In fact, a meta-analysis of more than 100 studies shows that teacher and parent training on ADHD can enhance the behavior of students, improve parent–teacher–student interactions and lessen disruptive behavior (Maughan, Christiansen, Jensen, Olympia, & Clark, 2005).

Helping Teachers Become Aware of the Nature
and Symptoms of ADHD

In addition to providing information about the legitimacy of ADHD as a disorder, school counselors can also increase teacher (and caregiver) awareness of the symptoms of ADHD (American Psychiatric Association, 2000) through individual consultation, team facilitation, or parent/teacher workshops. School counselors can help identify interventions that will likely improve the chances of school success for students diagnosed with ADHD. Over the last 25 years, concerned teachers have received in-service training, handbooks, and lists of strategies for teaching to students with ADHD. However, some teachers appear to be overwhelmed by the task of accommodating students with ADHD. There are a handful of specific strategies that are most likely to increase the likelihood that students with ADHD will be successful in the classroom. Examples of these types of accommodation strategies include:

- Allowing physical rearrangements in the classroom, such as preferential seating or opportunities for physical breaks in activity;
- Providing tips for teacher instruction, such as alternate grading methods (e.g., grades based on what has been completed or for marking correct and incorrect responses), or shortening the length of homework assignments;
- Allowing testing modifications such as oral exams, or allowing long exams to be taken in shorter segments; and
- Providing tips for home and school communication for students with ADHD, such as developing a of daily or weekly system for teachers and caregivers to communicate the student's progress.

    A more complete description of proven classroom interventions can be found at the Web site http://www.greatschools.net/articles/68/LD/Identifying-a-Learning-Difficulty/AD-HD-Basics.

Zentall (2006) suggested a three-way approach to helping students with ADHD maintain attention over time. The first approach is changing the child through a combination of medical and behavioral interventions. School counselors can provide direct service to students with ADHD through behavioral and cognitive behavioral interventions to help them. The second approach is changing the task the child is being asked to attend to by varying the length of the task or assignment, adjusting the level of attention needed to complete tasks throughout the day, and fluctuating the activity level involved in the completion of the task. For example, school counselors might help teachers understand the importance of cutting the number of homework math problems from 30 to 15 for students with ADHD, stopping every 20–30 minutes to have students think about the most important points from the previous lecture or discussion, and combining independent and group tasks to vary the level of attention required for successful participation. The third approach is changing the setting, such as providing a routine and limiting distractions. For example, a teacher might provide routine and consistent directions at the end of each class period regarding the recording of homework assignments in student planners. The routine might also include double-checking with another student seated nearby (who usually has the assignments recorded correctly) to make sure the student with ADHD has enough information recorded to complete the assignments at home. Another example would be moving the student's seat closer to the front of the class or away from the door to limit distractions. All students can benefit from these strategies; however, the strategies are critical for students with ADHD.

In addition to knowing what modifications can help improve academic and behavioral outcomes for students with ADHD, it is important to identify the interventions that have not been proven to be effective. School counselors may receive questions about these types of intervention as well. Research has not supported popularly held views that ADHD arises from excessive sugar intake, food additives, excessive viewing of television, or poor child management by parents (Barkley, 1998; Conners, 1980; Consensus Development Panel, 1985; Roth, & Drucker, 2008). While limiting sugar or monitoring television watching may be important to the overall health and well-being of children, they do not cause or cure ADHD. School counselors would not likely discourage parents from such strategies as part of a healthy lifestyle. However, it would be important for school counselors to advise parents regarding the research supporting the effectiveness of these types of interventions for *treating* ADHD.

Anticipating the Needs of Students with ADHD and Planning Appropriate Interventions

School counselors can also help teachers understand and anticipate the needs of students with ADHD and plan accordingly. Again, this need speaks to the legitimacy of the disorder. Take for example a color-blind high school student taking biology. The teacher plans an exam that involves labeling the parts of a frog using a color-coded system. The teacher knows the student will have difficulty completing the task and anticipates the need to create an accommodation. The teacher quickly devises a number-coded system so the student has an equal opportunity to complete the task. More often than not, teachers do not anticipate the needs of students with ADHD with the same certainty.

Accommodating the Needs of Students with ADHD

When teachers acknowledge ADHD as a legitimate disorder, are aware of the symptoms of the disorder along with appropriate accommodations, and are willing to anticipate the needs of students with ADHD, accommodating students' needs becomes a part of their overall teaching strategy. The school counselor is in a unique position to become familiar with students and families over time. The counselor can help create a context for each teacher related to what has worked for the student in the past, what progress has been made, and what strategies need to be altered. They may assist with the development of classroom accommodations or more formal 504 plans and Individual Education Plans

(IEPs) that become part of the daily teaching strategy (U.S. Department of Special Education Practice, 2006).

School counselors play a critical role in helping teachers reach the point of proactive accommodation. As previously mentioned, teachers have long had information and access to lists of intervention strategies for students with ADHD. Often it takes the efforts of other adults, such as school counselors and parents or caregivers, advocating for the needs and legitimacy of ADHD to create proactive learning environments in which students have improved chances of being successful.

CONSULTING WITH SCHOOL PSYCHOLOGISTS
AND MEDICAL PROFESSIONALS

An important school-based resource for counselors working with students with ADHD is the school psychologist. School counselors can work with school psychologists to determine if a student is exhibiting behaviors consistent with ADHD. The school psychologist is also the professional who will likely determine if learning disabilities also accompany or *cause* the observed behaviors. This is an important determination that can be difficult. For example, one school counselor was consulted about ADHD regarding a fourth grade student. The counselor observed the student during social studies lesson time, in which reading and comprehension were required. The student appeared to exhibit many of the off-task behaviors associated with ADHD and did not know how to respond when called upon. However, when the student was observed during the math lesson, she was on task, attentive, raised her hand, and upon review of her in-class practice assignment, it was clear she understood the content. After consultation with the school psychologist, it was suggested that a learning disability be explored as a first option since behaviors associated with ADHD were not consistent across academic settings, nor were they being reported at home. This collaborative approach with another school professional with knowledge of ADHD and other learning difficulties creates a solid base on which recommendations can be made to parents to seek medical consultation regarding ADHD.

When parents do decide to seek medical consultation, the medical professional will likely want input from teachers and other school personnel regarding the observed behaviors of the student they are diagnosing. Since there is no definitive test for ADHD, school-based observations are highly important components of the medical professionals' evaluations. Teachers are frequently asked to complete rating scales reflecting their observations of students suspected to have ADHD, such as the Conner's Rating Scale Revised (Conners, 2001) or the ADD–H Comprehensive Teacher's Rating Scale (Ullmann, Sleator, & Sprague, 1999). The Conner's Rating Scale Revised (CRS–R) is completed by parents and/or teachers to assist medical professionals by capturing observations of behaviors associated with ADHD. The ADD–H Comprehensive Teacher's Rating Scale (ACTeRS) is completed by teachers to assist in the diagnosis of ADHD.

The counselor is frequently asked to facilitate this collaborative process between school personnel and outside professionals in determining if ADHD is the appropriate diagnosis for a student.

Once a diagnosis of ADHD has been established, the school counselor can continue to be an important link as appropriate intervention strategies are determined. With parental consent, the school counselor can consult directly with medical professionals regarding changes in behavior, particularly if medication has been prescribed. While Ritalin (a methylphenidate) is one of the most widely studied medications prescribed to children, many other stimulant medications are also prescribed for children with ADHD. Other forms of methylphenidate, along with amphetamine-based medications (also stimulants), are often prescribed for children with ADHD. Amphetamine-based medications include Adderall and Dexedrine. Stimulants work by enhancing the brain's ability to inhibit itself, resulting in less distractibility and less impulsivity. Straterra is the only non-stimulant approved by the FDA for the treatment of ADHD and is categorized as an anti-depressant. It often takes trials of various doses or various medications to find what works for students diagnosed with ADHD who require medication. This is part of an ongoing process of finding the most effective combination of strategies for students with ADHD.

Writing for a Web site dedicated to helping the public understand learning disabilities and ADHD, Kidder (2002) provides a useful overview of the role of school-based and other helping and medical professionals and their ability to diagnose ADHD and prescribe medication. A more complete description of ADHD medications including names of medications, effects, duration of effects, pros, and precautions can be found on numerous reputable Web sites (e.g., http://www.ncpamd.com/adhd_and_medication.htm). Another good source for information on stimulant medications for ADHD can be found National Institutes of Health Web sites: http://www.nida.nih.gov/infofacts/ADHD.html and http://www.nimh.nih.gov/health/publications/attention-deficit-hyperactivity-disorder/medications.shtml

DIRECT SCHOOL COUNSELOR INTERVENTION

Shillingford et al. (2007) recommended that professional school counselors use an integrative approach to assist students with ADHD, one that combines cognitive-behavioral theory and systems thinking to direct interventions. Within this systemic context, counselors (1) become knowledgeable about their role in the identification and support of students with ADHD as well as their ethical and legal obligations in this regard; (2) act as consultants providing timely and pertinent information to parents/guardians and teachers; (3) follow children with ADHD (and their families) over time and assist them in using appropriate classroom interventions; and (4) provide direct service to students with ADHD through individual and small group work. The following interventions are some examples of school counselor-led programs aimed at helping students with ADHD understand and take responsibility for their disorder and provide various skills training aimed at improving academic and social outcomes.

The Journey

Webb and Myrick (2003) developed a six-week small group counseling intervention aimed at helping students with ADHD understand how symptoms of ADHD influence their "journey" in the world of education. It provides language and tools to help students become successful in school. The intervention is intended to empower students with ADHD and help them be more responsible for managing their actions. Session topics and key points include:

- Session 1: Beginning the Journey. Students participate in a map activity exploring various paths to a single destination. The connection is made to "school success" as the destination and that different kinds of learners sometimes need to take different paths.

- Session 2: Pack it Up. The counselor begins by rummaging through a bag or backpack looking for something that cannot be found, demonstrating the problems that can result from being disorganized. Some organizational strategies are introduced, demonstrated, and practiced using the students' own backpacks. Students talk about other places they might become more organized to help them on their "journey."

- Session 3: Stop Lights and Traffic Cops. Students take an imaginary "car ride" to heighten their awareness of the need to pay attention. Students relate to other times it is particularly important to pay attention. Students are introduced to and practice attending skills and strategies that can make paying attention and listening easier.

- Session 4: Using Road Signs as a Guide. Students identify common road signs that cue behavior, then think about what kinds of cues and reminders they might use to make learning easier.

- Session 5: Road Holes and Detours. Students brainstorm what could go wrong on a road trip that would make it difficult to reach their destination. Students then think about potential "school success" obstacles and brainstorm strategies for overcoming them. The counselor introduces selected cognitive behavioral strategies aimed at helping students with ADHD use detours to get around "road holes."

- Session 6: Roadside Help and Being Your Own Mechanic. Students consider skills they have learned up to this point that can be used to help them be more successful in school. As students become more empowered and responsible for their actions, they learn to recognize that sometimes more help is needed. The session also discusses medication as a necessary tool in the toolbox for some students with ADHD.

The six-week intervention is followed by monthly booster sessions to continue to help students monitor their further progress toward the goals they have set for themselves and to provide an opportunity to share successes.

Teaching Self-Monitoring Strategies

Studies suggest that teaching self-monitoring skills to students with ADHD improves their academic performance (e.g, Friedlander, Saddler, Frizzelle, & Graham, 2005; Shimabukuro, Prater, Jenkins, & Edelen-Smith, 1999). For example, Prater et al. (1999) reviewed the literature and investigated the effects of self-monitoring on academic performance and on-task behavior for students with ADHD and other learning disabilities. Their summary cited numerous studies that indicate self-monitoring procedures can be effective in helping students with mild disabilities improve their school performance. In their own study (Shimabukuro et al., 1999), middle school students were given structured amounts of time to complete assignments and correct their own work. Students also received teacher feedback regarding their performance. Students were instructed in self-monitoring and graphed their completion and accuracy percentages after each assignment. Students improved in the amount of work they were completing and the number of items they were getting correct in addition to being observed to be more on task by their teachers. Zentall (2006) also reviewed studies involving self-monitoring strategies and reported that 86% of the studies from school-based samples showed improved attention and behavioral outcomes.

School counselors can teach students how to monitor and graph their progress through individual or small group sessions. This can be helpful as the classroom teacher may not have the same opportunities to work with the student to teach the strategy. However, teachers are part of the collaborative process by providing students the opportunity to graph their completion and accuracy outcomes at the end of each class period and providing encouragement and feedback on a daily basis regarding student outcomes.

Working with High School Students

Schwiebert, Sealander, and Dennison (2002) have pulled together interventions particularly helpful for high school students with ADHD aimed at learning, relationship building, daily living, and transition to post-secondary pursuits. Again, these strategies can be taught through individual or small group sessions and cued by the classroom teacher. One example of the many learning strategies they describe was developed by Ellis and Lenz (1987). It involves the mnemonic "CANDO" to help students remember content information.

C   Create a list of items to be learned

A   Ask yourself if the list is complete

N   Note the main ideas and details by creating an map or diagram

D   Describe each component on your map and how they relate

O   Overlearn main points and build with details

School counselors can help students learn to use similar strategies to create organized frameworks for approaching learning. Strategies for managing daily living were also described by Schwiebert et al. (2002). One example involved strategies developed by Nadeau (1995) to help those with ADHD avoid under-stimulation. Nadeau suggested:

- Taking frequent breaks from any boring but necessary activity
- Mixing low interest and high interest activities
- Interacting with other people
- Engaging in physical exercise
- Creating challenges to increase interest
- Choosing a career with high intrinsic motivation

Stop and Think

Another curriculum developed for use with students diagnosed with ADHD is Philip Kendall's (1992) Stop and Think program. It lends itself well to work with impulsive students and fosters the acquisition of the problem-solving steps and rules for learning to STOP and THINK. Middle sessions shift to the application of problem-solving steps in social situations. The final sessions deal with the child's particular behavior problems and involve role playing of alternative solutions to specific problematic situations. The purpose here is to apply problem-solving steps to emotionally arousing situations. School counselors can collaborate with behavior specialists, teachers, and other school personnel who may be involved in the day to day education of students with ADHD to share Stop and Think concepts and language and to help cue students to use the problem-solving steps or encourage students to make appropriate choices.

SUMMARY

School counselors play an important role in helping parents, caregivers, and teachers identify and accommodate students with ADHD. They can provide direct service through individual and small group interventions. However, one of their most important roles may be affecting the attitudes of school personnel regarding the legitimacy of ADHD and the need to anticipate and accommodate students' needs just as they would do for any other students with identified disabilities. Counselors can help teachers recognize student strengths and encourage parents and teachers to include students in the treatment process. This inclusion and the idea that students with ADHD can make contributions to their own treatment reflect a recent shift toward a more positive approach in treating students with ADHD (Rief, 2005). This also empowers the student to become more responsible for his or her behavior. As Dr. Sam Goldstein (2005), a leading researcher in the field of ADHD, stated:

> Treatment planning (for ADHD) must not only include identifying strategies to manage problematic symptoms and behaviors but also finding strategies to build on what's right, to facilitate self-esteem, resilience, and a sense of self-efficacy. The discussion of treatment planning must focus equally on what is right as upon what is wrong. (p. 33)

TABLE 1.1   Additional Resources for Assisting Students with ADHD

- ADD Warehouse Web site: http://www.addwarehouse.com

- Attention Deficit Disorders Association (ADDA) Web site: http://add.org

- Centers for Disease Control and Prevention (CDC). (2009). *Attention-deficit/hyperactivity disorder (ADHD)*. Web site: http://www.cdc.gov/ncbddd/adhd/facts.html (amazing array of valuable information on all facets of ADHD)

- Children and Adults with ADHD (CHADD) Web site: http://www.chadd.org

- Council for Exceptional Children Web site: http://cec.sped.org/ (search "ADHD")

- Mental Health Association of America. Web site: http://www.nmha.org/ (covers emotional disorders in useful and readable language)

- National Institute of Mental Health (NIMH). *Mental health topics*. Web site: from http://www.nimh.nih.gov/health/topics/ (provides valuable general information)

- Dr. Barkley website: *About ADHD: A fact sheet by Dr. Barkley* http://www.russellbarkley.org/adhd-facts.htm

- Dr. Goldstein website: http://www.samgoldstein.com Medications chart Web site: http://www.webmd.com/solutions/adhd-and-your-child/adhd-medications-chart

- National Information Center for Children and Youth with Disabilities Web site: http://www.nichcy.org (Search "ADHD")

- National Institute of Mental Health Web site: http://www.help4adhd.org

- National Resource Center on AD/HD (NRC): A Program of CHADD (Children and Adults with Attention-Deficit/Hyperactivity Disorder) Web site: http://help4adhd.org/aboutus.cfm

- Schwab Foundation web site: http://www.schwablearning.org

- US Office of Special Education Practice Web site: http://www.ed.gov/about/offices/list/osers/osep/index.html (search "ADHD")

School counselors can help parents and school professionals focus on what is "right" about students like Caleb. They can work directly through individual and group work or indirectly through consultation with parents and teachers to build on the student's strengths as part of the intervention process. Readers are encouraged to consult Table 1.1 for additional information regarding the identification and treatment of students with ADHD.

REFERENCES

American Psychiatric Association. (2000). *Diagnostic and statistical manual of mental disorders* (Text Rev., 4th ed.). Washington, D.C.: Author.

Barkley, R. A. (1998). Attention deficit hyperactivity disorder. *Scientific American, 3,* 279–285.

Barkley, R. A. (2006). *Attention deficit hyperactivity disorder: A handbook for diagnosis and treatment* (3rd ed.). New York: Guilford. Available on line at http://www.russellbarkley.org/images/BarkleyCh01.pdf

Barkley, R. A., Cook, E., Diamond, A., Zametkim, A., Thapar, A., & Teeter, A., et al. (2002). International consensus statement on ADHD. *Clinical Child and Family Psychology Review, 5*, 89–111. Retrieved May 25, 2009, from http://www. russellbarkley.org/images/Consensus%202002.pdf

Barkley, R. A., Fischer, M., Edelbrock, C., & Smallish, L. (1990). The adolescent outcome of hyperactive children diagnosed by research criteria I: An 8–year prospective follow-up study. *Journal of the American Academy of Child and Adolescent Psychiatry, 29*, 546–557.

Biederman, J., Farone, S., & Lapey, K. (1992). Comorbidity of diagnosis in attention deficit hyperactivity disorder. In G. Weiss (Ed.), *Child and adolescent psychiatric clinics of North America: Attention deficit hyperactivity disorder* (pp. 355–360). Philadelphia, PA: Saunders.

Centers for Disease Control and Prevention (CDC). (2009). *Attention-deficit/hyperactivity disorder (ADHD).* Retrieved May 28, 2008, from http://www.cdc.gov/ncbddd/adhd/facts.html

Conners, C. K. (1980). *Food additives and hyperactive children.* New York: Plenum.

Conners, C. K. (2001). *Conners' rating scales–revised technical manual.* North Tonawanda, New York: Multi Health Systems.

Consensus Development Panel. (1985). *Defined diets and childhood hyperactivity: National Institute of Health consensus statement.* Bethesda, MD: National Institute of Health.

Doll, B., & Cummings, J. A. (2008). *Transforming school mental health services population-based approaches to promoting the competency and wellness of children.* Thousand Oaks, CA: Corwin.

DuPaul, G., & Stoner, G. (1994). *ADHD in the schools: Assessment and intervention strategies.* New York: Guilford.

Ellis, E., & Lenz, B. (1987). A component analysis of effective learning for LD students. *Learning Disabilities Focus, 2*, 94–107.

Friedlander, B. D., Saddler, B., Frizzelle, R., & Graham, S. (2005). Self-monitoring of attention versus self-monitoring of academic performance: Effects among students with ADHD in the general education classroom. *Journal of Special Education, 39*, 145–156.

Goldstein, S. (2005) *Update on ADHD.* Retrieved on May 28, 2009, from http://www. samgoldstein.com/node/94

Goldstein, S., & Goldstein, M. (1998). *Managing attention deficit hyperactivity disorder in children: A guide for practitioners* (2nd ed.). New York: Wiley.

Gordon, M. (1993). *I would if I could: A teenager's guide to ADHD/hyperactivity.* DeWitt, NY: GSI Publications.

Harnett, D. N., Nelson, J. M., & Rinn, A. N. (2004). Gifted or ADHD? The possibilities of misdiagnosis. *Roeper Review, 26*, 73–76.

Kendall, P. (1992). *Stop and think workbook.* Philadelphia, PA: Workbook Publishing.

Kidder, K. R. (2002). *Who can diagnosis LD and/or ADHD.* Retrieved May 28, 2009, from http://www.ldonline.org/article/6027

Maughan, D. R., Christiansen, E., Jenson, W. R., Olympia, D., & Clark, E. (2005). Behavioral parent training as a treatment for externalizing behavior disorders: A meta-analysis. *School Psychology Review, 34*, 267–286.

McKinney, J., Montague, M., & Hocutt, A. (1993). Educational assessment of children with attention deficit disorder. *Exceptional Children, 60*, 125–131.

Nadeau, K. (1995). Life management skills for adults with ADD. In K.Nadeau (Eds.), *A comprehensive guide to attention deficit disorder in adults* (pp. 191–217). New York: Bruner/Mazel.

Rief, S. F. (2005). *How to reach and teach children with ADD/ADHD: Practical techniques, strategies, and interventions.* San Francisco, CA: Josey-Bass.

Roth, M., & Drucker, R. (2008). Nutritional requirements for children with special needs. *Exceptional Parent, 38*, 24–27.

Schwiebert, V., Sealander, K., & Dennison, J. (2002). Strategies for counselors working with high school students with attention deficit hyperactivity disorder. *Journal of Counseling and Development, 80*, 3–10.

Shillingford, M. A., Lambie, G., & Walter, S. M. (2007). An integrative, cognitive-behavioral, systemic approach to working with students diagnosed with attention deficit hyperactive disorder. *Professional School Counseling, 11*, 105–112.

Shimabukuro, S., Prater, M., Jenkins, A., & Edelen-Smith, P. (1999). The effects of self-monitoring of academic performance on students with learning disabilities and ADD/ADHD. *Education and Treatment of Children 22*, 397–414.

Ullmann, R., Sleator, E., & Sprague, R. (1999). *The ADD–H Comprehensive Teacher's Rating Scale (ACTeRS)* (2nd ed.). Champaign, IL: MetriTech Inc.

US Department of Education. (2001). *No Child Left Behind Act of 2001.* Retrieved May 28, 2009, from http://www.ed.gov/nclb/landing.jhtml

US Department of Education Office for Civil Rights. (2009). *Protecting students with disabilities.* Retrieved May 28, 2009, from http://www.ed.gov/about/offices/list/ocr/504faq.html

US Office of Special Education Practice. (2006). *Teaching children with attention deficit hyperactivity disorder: Instructional strategies and practices.* Washington, DC: Author. Retrieved May 28, 2009, from http://www.ed.gov/rschstat/research/pubs/adhd/adhd-teaching-2006.pdf

Visser, S. N., Lesesne, C. A., & Perou, R. (2007). National estimates and factors associated with medication treatment for childhood attention-deficit/hyperactivity disorder. *Pediatrics, 119*, S99–S106.

Webb, L. D., & Myrick, R. D. (2003). A group counseling intervention for children with attention deficit hyperactivity disorder. *Professional School Counseling, 7*, 108–115.

Zentall, S. (2006). *ADHD and education: Foundations, characteristics, methods, and collaboration.* Upper Saddle River, NJ: Pearson Merrill.

Chapter 2

Externalizing Behavior Disorders

Supporting Students with Aggression and Violent Tendencies

KERRY B. BERNES, JENNIFER I. BERNES AND
ANGELA D. BARDICK

**University of Lethbridge,
Lethbridge, Alberta, Canada,
Registered Psychologist,
and Registered Psychologist**

Children and youth often engage in externalizing behaviors as they begin to explore and understand boundaries, form a sense of identity, and seek to understand social norms and values. However, some students may present with externalizing behaviors that are of significant concern to schools, especially bullying other students, harassment, threats, and other forms of violence. A vast number of school-based programs have been designed to prevent bullying and violence in schools, and seek to teach students about tolerance, acceptance, and developing a positive school environment. Regrettably, many of these programs tend to be reactive rather than proactive (Kauffman, 1999), and often do not appropriately identify and assess individual static, dynamic, and contextual factors that contribute to these externalizing behaviors. The professional school counselor has a significant role to play in assessing and intervening when a student displays serious externalizing behaviors. This chapter provides school counselors with a framework for identifying, assessing, and intervening when students present with externalizing behaviors that eventually develop into a disorder. The primary goal is to illustrate how a comprehensive assessment of school-age children's externalizing behaviors is essential to developing specific, individualized, and well-conceptualized interventions. The use of family interventions in assisting students with highly disruptive behaviors, including students with behavior disorders, is overviewed in chapter 7.

The case study of TJ, an adolescent with some challenging externalizing behaviors, is first described. A description of externalizing behaviors, a framework for identifying and assessing externalizing behaviors (including risk and targeted violence) using standardized assessment instruments appropriate for use by school counselors will follow. Finally, the case study of TJ will be used to illustrate how comprehensive assessment leads to concise and individualized plans for intervention.

TJ: A School-Based Case Study

TJ, a 14 year old, has been described as a "problem child" and a "behavior concern" by his teachers since kindergarten. TJ's school file indicated that up until the fifth grade, he appeared to have made average academic progress; however, his behavior in school interfered with his social progress. He was often the instigator of physical fights on the playground and was disruptive in the classroom. He appeared to have little empathy with his peers. TJ would behave in a very immature manner with peers, not appearing to notice their displays of disapproval. Although TJ craved his teacher's praise and could be very caring and considerate, he would become defiant and defensive when he was corrected for his off-task behaviors and frequent peer conflicts in the classroom. On one occasion TJ inappropriately fondled a female student in an aggressive manner and attacked another peer on the playground during recess. TJ had engaged in three incidents of minor vandalism in his school. On three occasions in the past year, TJ graphically described the violent actions he could inflict on teachers and peers. Statements such as "I know where you live, I will break in and kill you in your sleep" led people to be fearful of him. When school administrators attempted to resolve the issue with him, TJ would describe his behavior as out of his control due to "my ADHD" and "trauma and anxiety." Individuals working with TJ became frustrated with his resistance to change his perception and his continued explanations of "I have this problem, I can't help it, I get real mad and freak out when people make me mad and tell me what to do."

TJ's externalizing behaviors present significant challenges for the professional school counselor. To develop an effective intervention plan for addressing TJ's aggressive behavior and threats to harm his peers and teachers, the school counselor will first need an understanding of externalizing behaviors, a framework for effectively assessing TJ's level of risk, and knowledge of how to use the results of the assessment to develop effective interventions.

CHARACTERISTICS OF EXTERNALIZING
BEHAVIORS AND BEHAVIOR DISORDERS

Externalizing behaviors reflect a child's negative behavior on the external environment, whereas internalizing behaviors reflect problems on a child's psychological, or internal, environment (Troop-Gordon & Ladd, 2005). Generally, externalizing behaviors may be placed on a continuum that ranges from mild behaviors such as teasing, name-calling, bullying, and other forms of intimidation and harassment to severe behaviors such as physical fights and shootings (Hernández & Seem, 2004; Smith & Sandhu, 2004). Children of any age may demonstrate a number of externalizing behaviors without being explicitly identified as high risk. Unfortunately, it can be difficult to differentiate between normal childhood behaviors and those that indicate a serious risk for violence. It is therefore important to monitor students' externalizing behaviors carefully, because we cannot predict which students will continue to demonstrate increasingly severe externalizing behaviors (Troop-Gordon & Ladd) and which students' behaviors may resolve over time (Bongers, Koot, van der Ende, & Verhulst, 2004; Morgan, Farkas, & Wu, 2009).

There are links between young children's aggressive behaviors (e.g., hitting, kicking, verbal insults and threats), adolescent violence (e.g., homicide, assault; Conduct Problems Prevention Research Group, 1999; Singer & Flannery, 2000), and adult substance abuse, criminality, and domestic violence (Farrington, 2005; Ross, 1996). Children and youth who engage in a number of externalizing behaviors with increasing severity, frequency, and intensity over time may demonstrate an increased risk for violence. An ongoing pattern of aggressive and externalizing behaviors in younger students requires early identification, assessment and intervention (Morgan et al.). Gone untreated students with internalizing (see Chapter 3) and externalizing behavior problems are at a greater risk for a variety of negative long-term behavior problems, including poor academic achievement and failure at school (Lopes, 2007; Niesyn, 2009), a low socio-economic level, chronic or extended unemployment, and criminal behavior leading to incarceration (Morgan et al.).

Hyperactivity, aggression, and delinquency are considered the three primary constructs of externalizing behavior disorders (Liu, 2004; Merrill, 2008). According to the *Diagnostic and Statistical Manual of Mental Disorders–Text Revision* (DSM–IV–TR; American Psychiatric Association [APA], 2000), externalizing behaviors fall under the category of Attention-Deficit and Disruptive Behavior Disorders, which include Attention Deficit Hyperactivity Disorder (ADHD), Oppositional Defiant Disorder (ODD), and Conduct Disorder (CD). Students with ADHD, especially those with high impulsivity, often demonstrate externalizing behaviors (Webster et al., 1997). Students with ODD often demonstrate even more severe externalizing behaviors. According to the DSM–IV–TR, a diagnosis of ODD includes a "pattern of negativistic, hostile, and defiant behavior" (APA, 2000, p. 102). Students diagnosed with CD often present with the most severe externalizing behaviors. According to the DSM–IV–TR, a diagnosis of CD includes a combination of (A) aggression to people or animals, (B) destruction of property, (C) lying or theft, or (D) any violation of rules (APA, 2000). However, students with externalizing behaviors do not necessarily require a specific diagnosis before school counselors or other adults recognize the need for identification, assessment, and intervention. If a student is eventually labeled with an externalizing behavior disorder such as conduct disorder (CD), in school the student would be classified as having an emotional and behavioral disorder (EBD; Niesyn, 2009).

Prevalence and Etiology

Because of comorbidity issues (overlapping disorders within the same student), researchers find it challenging to estimate the prevalence rate for externalizing behavior problems in school-age children and youth. Although Merrill (2008, p. 276) suggests that "externalizing problems tend to be quite common," typically the prevalence rate is disaggregated based on which externalizing behavior disorder subtype one is addressing. For example, ADHD, an externalizing disorder, occurs more frequently in boys than girls (see Chapter 1), with [overall prevalence rates] of ADHD ranging from approximately 4:1 to 9:1 (Merrill). Similarly, CD prevalence rates vary from 4% to 8% in the entire school-age population, with boys again outnumbering girls on an average of 3:1.

The potential causes of externalizing disorders are hotly debated (see Merrill, 2008, for summary). Etiological perspectives range from dysfunctional social learning to neurobiological explanations. Needless to say, the causes are multidimensional and school counselors should not latch on to one preferred theory over others.

Identifying Externalizing Behaviors

Teachers are often the first to identify students with externalizing behaviors because children spend the majority of their time in the classroom (Cullerton-Sen & Crick, 2005). Thus, behavioral referrals to school counselors are most likely to come from individual teachers and school-wide screening processes (Walker, Cheney, Stage, Blum, & Horner, 2005). However, other methods such as mapping, documenting teacher and student reports, and observations are recommended to assist school counselors in further identifying students who present with externalizing behaviors (see Merrill, 2008, for a good overview).

Mapping   Mapping methods are useful to help school professionals identify students with externalizing behaviors in addition to identifying locations that may be more prone to violence, such as school playgrounds, auditoriums, hallways, cafeterias, sport fields, and routes to and from school (Astor, Benbenishty, & Meyer, 2004). Mapping methods allow "students and teachers to convey their personal theories about why specific locations and times in their schools are more dangerous" (Astor et al., p. 47). Mapping is also helpful to identify students, or groups of students, who may be more likely to engage in aggressive behaviors in these locations.

Student and Teacher Reports   Student and teacher reports of externalizing behavior can also provide valuable information about children's externalizing behaviors (Anderson-Butcher, Newsome, & Nay, 2003; Astor et al., 2004). Any reports of externalizing behavior (from teachers or from students) should be documented in a student's individual file. This provides a record of any problematic behaviors, and can be useful for tracking patterns of behavior over time.

Peer reports should be considered sources of valuable information about students with externalizing behaviors, as a student's peers may be more aware of certain behaviors and issues than teachers (Mishna & Alaggia, 2005; Worthen, Borg, & White, 1993). For example, peers may be more aware of other students' property violations (e.g., stealing and vandalism) or drug and alcohol use than adults.

Observations   Observations produce information regarding students' behaviors and circumstances that contribute to externalizing behaviors. However, they only provide information regarding specific incidents and generally do not correlate well over time. Observations may consist of unstructured observations and informal conversations with teachers and/or students. Structured observational methods, such as direct observations or the use of standardized forms, may also be used to examine behavioral patterns (Crothers & Levinson, 2004), although these may be more costly in terms of money and time. Ideal settings for observing students' behaviors are areas where there tend to be less adult direction, such as sport fields, school playgrounds, lunch rooms, restrooms, busses, locker rooms, and physical education classes (Crothers & Levinson).

Mapping, documenting teacher and student reports, and observations may be used as tools for identifying externalizing behaviors. However, even with the identification of externalizing behaviors, it is difficult for professional school counselors to plan effective interventions for students who demonstrate these behaviors without a thorough understanding of the individual static, dynamic, and contextual factors that may contribute to the child's behaviors. A framework for conducting a comprehensive assessment of student behaviors and the context in which they occur is next discussed.

Assessing Externalizing Behaviors

The purpose of assessment is to help answer questions regarding a student's behavioral concerns, potential risk to self or others, cognitive ability, adaptive functioning, placement considerations, and educational or vocational planning in order to inform recommendations for intervention. A behavioral assessment can specifically answer the questions "How severe are the child's behaviors?," "Why is this student behaving in this manner?," and "What can be done to help this student individually, at home, and at school?" More importantly, assessment provides valuable information to inform future planning for the student.

Some students may demonstrate externalizing behaviors that require further investigation, thus necessitating the use of more formal assessment approaches. The informed consent of the student's parents and/or guardians is essential to obtain before proceeding with a behavioral assessment. A variety of assessment techniques are necessary to obtain a balanced perspective of the student's externalizing behaviors and avoid incorrectly or inappropriately using information.

A comprehensive assessment of externalizing behaviors in school-age children includes the use of standardized assessment instruments, behavioral observations in different settings (e.g., home, school), and interviews with multiple informants (e.g., teachers, parents, peers, police, family physician, and anyone who has worked with the child). Some students, like TJ in our case study, may present with more serious and complex externalizing behaviors, which may require an overall assessment of risk using a Structured Judgment Approach to risk assessment (Borum, Bartel, & Forth, 2003). In addition to an overall assessment of risk, some students, like TJ in our case study, may present as a possible threat to others and also require a targeted violence risk assessment. Careful assessment, thorough documentation, and professional consultation are recommended in order to reduce liability (Ash, 2002), demonstrate competence and accountability, and determine effective interventions. Moreover, Bernes and Bardick (2007) provide a practical framework for school counselors to follow when conducting adolescent violence risk assessments. Some of the suggestions made below reflect this assessment scaffolding.

Multi-Disciplinary Team   Ideally, the assessment of a student's externalizing behaviors should be implemented by a multi-disciplinary team made up of school counselors, school administrators, teachers, law enforcement personnel, social workers and psychologists who are trained in behavioral assessment. A designated team leader, generally the individual most trained in behavioral assessment, should be responsible for ensuring that students who demonstrate externalizing behavior be assessed. The use of a multi-disciplinary assessment team is important to reduce liability, inform the assessment, and engage in best practices for behavioral assessment, especially with students who present with extreme externalizing behaviors or who may be at risk for harming others.

Assessment Process

Based on the student's presenting concerns, a comprehensive assessment using standardized assessment instruments, risk assessment, and targeted violence risk assessment may be needed. First, the parents/guardians need to be notified of the need for an assessment, and the multi-disciplinary team will determine who should administer the assessment instruments, conduct interviews, and gather all relevant records (school, medical, a child or family welfare office, law enforcement personnel, etc.).

Family and Medical History   Often, a child's family and medical histories are unknown to the school. However, knowledge of a child's family background and medical history can provide some important contextual information regarding the child's current behavior. For example, in the case of TJ, family and medical histories revealed a background of physical abuse, trauma, inconsistent guardianship, recent loss of an adoptive family, and several psychiatric diagnoses (specifically, Reactive Attachment Disorder, Attention Deficit Hyperactivity Disorder, Generalized Anxiety Disorder, and Post Traumatic Stress Disorder), which provided a context for TJ's current behaviors. Although not every student may have experienced a traumatic family situation or have specific psychiatric diagnoses, this information is important for better understanding the context for the student's behavior.

School History   Social and/or academic difficulties in school may also contribute to a student's externalizing behaviors. In the case of TJ, school records indicated that he did not have academic difficulties, but that he had had difficulty getting along with his peers since kindergarten. A recent psycho-educational assessment revealed that he had significant strengths in performance abilities and a slight weakness in verbal abilities. These results indicated that TJ was functioning within age- and grade-level expectations and that any problems he might be experiencing in class were not related to deficits in his potential for academic achievement. A psycho-educational assessment may not be needed in every behavioral assessment, but an assessment of a student's cognitive and academic functioning may provide useful information for further informing intervention plans if academic difficulties are suspected.

Interviews   Interviews with a variety of sources provide further insight into a student's behaviors and the motivations for those behaviors. It is important include the perspectives of multiple individuals when assessing externalizing behaviors in students to obtain a clear picture, as behaviors may fluctuate in severity in different locations and in the presence different individuals (Achenbach, Krukowski, Dumenci, & Ivanova, 2005). Interviews with the student, parents, caregivers, teachers, other school personnel, family physicians, peers, and any other individuals who have worked with the child (e.g., a counselor, social worker, law enforcement personnel) are recommended to obtain insights into the child's behavior as well as to cross-check information (Cormier, 1994).

Cornell et al.'s (2004) decision-tree model was designed for use when conducting interviews regarding school threat assessments, and may provide a framework for conducting interviews regarding student's externalizing behaviors. All individuals involved with the student should be interviewed with a similar set of questions in order to verify information. Information about the behavior is gathered through asking the student a series of questions about the behavior (e.g., what happened, what the student intended by the behavior, any prior history of conflict, relationship with the victim(s), how the student perceives others to feel about the behavior, reasons for the behavior, and future intentions). The context in which the behavior occurred must also be examined, because contextual information may alter the seriousness of the behavior. Other topics that are important to address include mental health status, current level of stress, family relations, access to weapons, exposure to violence, and previous involvement in aggressive behaviors.

In TJ's case, an individual interview revealed that he did not trust adults or his peers, did not feel in control of his life, and was experiencing a lack of attachment and meaning. He revealed a history of self-harming behaviors (such as cutting) and previous suicide attempts. TJ believed he had strengths in sports, computers, drama and some school subjects, and that involvement with a community recreational basketball league was enjoyable. Interviews with his foster family, teachers, and community social worker revealed early involvement in both violent and non-violent offenses, anger management difficulties, and serious social deficits.

Standardized Assessment Instruments The American School Counselor Association (ASCA, 2004) recommends that professional school counselors "utilize assessment measures within the scope of practice for school counselors" (p. 2). There are several standardized assessment instruments that are appropriate for use by professional school counselors with graduate training in assessment, although it is beyond the scope of this chapter to provide a comprehensive description of each of these instruments. Rather, examples of commonly used instruments appropriate for a comprehensive behavioral assessment are provided in Table 2.1. For additional information on useful tools, see Merrill (2008, Chapter 9).

A comprehensive assessment of externalizing behaviors often includes a combination of appropriate assessment tools, depending on the age of the student and the severity of the presenting behaviors (Morgan et al., 2009). In TJ's case, a full battery of the assessment instruments cited in Table 2.1 were administered, including an overall assessment of behavior (BASC–2), a measure of depression (BDI–II), a measure of hopelessness (BHS), a suicide measure (SPS), and clinical measure (MACI), as well as a risk assessment (SAVRY) and a targeted violence risk assessment. The assessment instruments provided the following overview of TJ's current behavioral difficulties:

1. On the BASC–2, TJ had clinically significant scores on aggression, anxiety, attention problems, conduct problems, hyperactivity, and social skills.
2. On the BDI–II, TJ described himself as having severe symptoms of depression.
3. On the BHS, TJ described himself as having moderate feelings of hopelessness.
4. On the SPS (measure of potential for suicide), some potential for suicide was indicated.
5. The MACI interpretive report described TJ as anticipating rejection from others and thus acting out behaviorally; feeling confused and lost; having strong feelings of rejection, anger, and self-doubt; and having major difficulties with peer relationships.

These results are important to provide a psychological context for TJ's behaviors. As seen by these results, a child who is frustrated, confused, depressed,

T A B L E 2.1 Recommended Standardized Assessment Instruments for Assessing Externalizing Behaviors in School-age Children and Youth

Name of Instrument	Author	Age	Purpose	Description
Child Behavior Checklist for Ages 6–18 (CBCL/6-18)	Achenbach and Rescorla (2001)	6 to 18	Measures internalizing and externalizing behaviors	Uses information from student, parents/ caregivers, and teachers to provide descriptions of students' behaviors
Behavior Assessment System for Children, Second Edition (BASC–2)	Reynolds and Kamphaus (2004)	6 to 18	Measures internalizing and externalizing behaviors	Uses information from student, parents/ caregivers, and teachers to provide descriptions of students' behaviors
Children's Depression Inventory (CDI)	Kovaks (2001)	7 to 17	Measures symptoms of depression	27 self-report items that measures negative mood, interpersonal problems, ineffectiveness, anhedonia, and negative self-esteem
Beck Depression Inventory, Second Edition (BDI–II)	Beck, Steer, and Brown (1996)	13 and older	Measures severity of depressive symptoms	21 self-report items that measures symptoms such as sadness, pessimism, guilt, social withdrawal, and suicidal ideation
Beck Hopelessness Scale (BHS)	Beck and Steer (1993)	13 and older	Measures severity of feelings of hopelessness	18 self-report items

Instrument	Author (Year)	Age	Purpose	Description
Suicide Probability Scale (SPS)	Cull and Gill (1988)	14 and older	Measure of suicide potential	36 self-report items that measure presence and intensity hopelessness, suicidal ideation, negative self-evaluation and hostility
Millon Adolescent Clinical Inventory (MACI)	Millon (1993)	13 to 19	Psychological evaluation of adolescents	Elevated scores on self-report items are indicative of increasing probability of psychological problems; must be administered by a psychologist
Early Assessment Risk List for Boys (EARL–20B)	Augimeri, Koegl, Webster, and Levene, (2001)	Under 12 (boys)	Assessing risk factors associated with violence	Coordinates and evaluates information obtained from rating scales, interviews, self-reports, police records, direct observations, and standardized assessment instruments to provide a comprehensive assessment of children's risk for violence
Early Assessment Risk List for Girls (EARL–21G)	Levene et al. (2001)	Under 12 (girls)	Same as above	Same as above
The Structured Assessment of Violence and Risk in Youth (SAVRY)	Borum et al. (2003)	13 to 17	Assessing factors associated with risk for violence	Uses a rating scale to assess Historical, Social/Contextual, and Individual risk factors in addition to Protective factors to provide a comprehensive assessment of adolescent risk for violence

hopeless, hostile, self-defeating, aggressive, and feels rejected by others is certain to demonstrate some serious externalizing behaviors.

Risk Assessment A Structured Professional Judgment approach to risk assessment (Borum et al., 2003) is the most recent approach to assessing risk in children, adolescents, and adults. This approach to risk assessment examines a number of factors associated with risk in youth, such as historical factors, clinical and situational factors, and risk management factors (Webster, Douglas, Eaves, & Hart, 1997). Assessment of risk in adolescents also emphasizes dynamic and contextual risk factors, such as peer delinquency, peer rejection, poor parental management, and community disorganization (Borum et al.). Suicidal ideation must also be assessed, as one cannot be sure if a violent individual will harm the self or others (Cameron, 2000). Frick (2004) asserts that "the number of risk factors present is more important than the type of risk factor" (p. 824). Thus, the accumulation of risk factors is considered to be a stronger indication of potential for violence.

An examination of all of the associated risk factors, in addition to an examination of protective factors (e.g., a positive attitude toward intervention and authority, prosocial involvement, strong social support, strong attachments and bonds, strong commitment to school, resilient personality traits; Borum et al., 2003) are important components of a risk assessment. The manuals recommended for use by school counselors for conducting risk assessments in children and adolescents are summarized in Table 2.1.

Using the SAVRY, TJ was assessed at a moderate to high level across most risk factors. Specifically, TJ had a history of witnessing and being involved in violent acts from a young age, significant peer rejection, recent loss of adoptive family, diagnosis of ADHD and PTSD, and a lack of important protective factors. Although an assessment of general risk provides an overview of areas for intervention, an assessment of targeted violence risk is important to determine the potential for harm to others.

Targeted violence risk assessments are necessary to respond to any student's threat to harm others. If a student presents as an immediate risk for a violent act, parents and guardians should be notified immediately. In the case of violence risk assessment, the welfare of the student and other individuals takes priority over confidentiality (Capuzzi, 2002). If parents or guardians do not provide consent for a targeted violence risk assessment, referral to a child welfare service may be necessary.

Targeted violence risk assessments are very similar to suicide risk assessments. Similar questions apply, with a focus on ideation, plans, mood disorders (e.g., depression), substance use disorders, hopelessness, intention to die (or to kill), and lethality of means. Just as the information obtained from a suicide assessment can lead the school counselor to a determination of the degree of risk and targets for intervention (i.e., taking away the means, contracting, counseling, hospitalization, etc.; Capuzzi, 2002), a targeted violence risk assessment also informs degree of risk and can indicate targets for intervention. The primary question in the case of a targeted violence risk assessment is whether the student is "… on a pathway toward a violent act and if so how fast he or she is moving and where could one intervene?" (Borum & Reddy, 2001, p. 377).

Borum and Reddy (2001) developed the acronym ACTION to guide professionals in considering six areas of inquiry when conducting targeted violence risk assessments. ACTION stands for: (1) Attitudes that Support or Facilitate Violence, (2) Capacity, (3) Thresholds Crossed, (4) Intent, (5) Other's Reactions and Responses, and (6) Non-Compliance with Risk Reduction Interventions. Table 2.2 provides an overview of the ACTION acronym with specific questions for school counselors to answer in order to arrive at a determination of risk for targeted violence.

The ACTION (Borum & Reddy, 2001) acronym was used to assess TJ's risk for committing a violent act. Under the category of *Attitudes that Support or Facilitate Violence*, TJ clearly described to previous caregivers, school administrators, and the school counselor that the majority of the individuals he has assaulted "deserved it." TJ also admitted to hitting people or damaging things when angry. Under the category of *Capacity*, TJ had the physical ability to cause harm and displayed the physical ability to injure others even when he was restrained. Under the category of *Thresholds Crossed*, TJ had not taken any of the steps necessary to follow through on his threats, although his diagnosis of ADHD placed him at considerable risk for an impulsive act of violence. Under the category of *Intent*, TJ stated full intent and appeared to mean it in the heat of the moment. However, TJ did not appear to be making any movement to acquiring means, thus making his risk for a violent act more likely to be driven by impulse as opposed to planned. Under the *Other's Reactions and Responses* category, peers did not support his behaviors because they perceived his verbal and aggressive outbursts as being immature. Paid caregivers discouraged his belief system, and he felt guilty for his actions around his former adoptive family. The *Non-Compliance with Risk Reduction Interventions* category described TJ as being willing to prevent or avoid a violent act with those he felt close to (e.g., his former adoptive mother). In this case, the targeted violence risk assessment indicated that although TJ clearly had the capacity to commit a violent act, and had made threats to harm others, the threats appeared to be an impulsive reaction to an immediate situation rather than a planned premeditated intent to do harm.

As can be seen by the assessment procedure, a comprehensive assessment can identify a number of areas that require both immediate intervention (e.g., targeted violence) and long-term intervention. A comprehensive assessment can be used to assist a multi-disciplinary team in developing a concise intervention plan for helping students with externalizing behaviors mitigate risk and manage their behaviors more appropriately.

RECOMMENDATIONS FOR SCHOOL COUNSELING
PRACTICE—INTERVENTIONS

Individual, family, school, and community interventions often arise from a comprehensive assessment. Effective recommendations for intervention with students who demonstrate externalizing behaviors generally focus on the following categories: behavior management, counseling/therapeutic intervention, and educational/

T A B L E 2.2 **Targeted Violence Risk Assessment: Description of the ACTION Acronym**

ACTION Acronym	Description	Screening Questions
Attitudes that support or facilitate violence	Does the individual believe that the use of violence is justified under certain circumstances?	Has the individual hit people or damaged things when he or she is angry? Do you worry that the individual might physically hurt someone? Has there been a time when the individual has hurt someone (e.g., kicking, hitting, slapping, pushing, shoving, or grabbing?) Has the individual ever threatened anyone with a weapon?
Capacity	Does the individual have the capacity or means to carry out the type of violent act that he or she has threatened?	Does the individual have the physical and intellectual capabilities to carry out the act? Does the individual have access to means (weapons or materials necessary to follow through with the violent act)? Does the individual have access to the target(s)? Does the individual have the opportunity to commit the act?
Thresholds Crossed	What has the individual done in order to enact the plan, such as any attack-related behaviors or any behaviors that require breaking laws and/or school rules?	What steps has the individual followed in order to enact the plan? Has the individual acquired means? Has the individual broken any laws or school rules?
Intent	What is the connection between the individual's thoughts and intentions to commit the act?	Does the individual have thoughts or intentions to commit a violent act? How specific is the plan? Is the individual making any movement to acquiring the means? Does the individual believe that he or she has no other available options or that he or she has nothing to lose?
Other's Reactions and Responses	How have other individuals responded to the individual's plans?	Has the individual communicated with anyone about his or her plans for violence? How does the individual report that others have responded? Have others discouraged, condemned the ideas, offered no judgment, supported or escalated the violent ideas, or even facilitated the movement from idea to action? Are others concerned he or she may do it?
Non-Compliance with Risk Reduction Interventions	What is the individual's willingness, motivation, and history of engaging in risk reduction interventions?	Is the individual motivated to prevent or avoid a violent act? Is the individual willing to participate in interventions to reduce or mitigate risk? Does the individual have a history of complying with risk reduction efforts? Does the individual possess enough insight to understand or appreciate the severity of his or her own disorder (if one exists), need for treatment, and/or the potential for violence?

28

SOURCE:

vocational planning. Recommendations should not only focus on helping the student modify their behaviors, but also help professional school counselors, teachers, and parents and caregivers change the contexts in which the student's behaviors occur in order to improve functioning in different environments.

Behavior Management

Behavior management is an important component of treatment for students who demonstrate behavior disorders. The following are general behavior management recommendations, which may vary according to each student's individual needs:

- Students with psychiatric diagnoses (e.g., ADHD, ODD, CD, depression, anxiety, etc.) will require ongoing monitoring by a child psychiatrist and family physician to assess and monitor appropriate medications.

- Students with externalizing behaviors will require consistent and appropriate discipline with consequences for both positive and negative behaviors. Therefore, support and training for caregivers and all teachers and school support staff is recommended to deal with each student's unique needs and learn how to consistently set firm but caring boundaries while simultaneously reinforcing positive behaviors.

- Students may benefit from instruction in self-calming strategies (e.g., in TJ's case, he found intense physical exercise as well as drawing to be calming).

- Students may be taught to self-monitor their behaviors and request time-outs when they believe they need time to calm down. (e.g., in TJ's case, the metaphor of an "anger thermometer" was helpful for him to self-monitor his level of anger on a scale of 1 to 10, and request a time-out in a quiet place when his "anger temperature" reached the level 5).

- Students with severe aggressive behaviors may respond well to having a quiet room set aside in which to de-escalate their feelings of agression.

- Students may benefit from processing any behavioral outbursts in a caring, non-judgmental manner with a supportive adult after the outburst event has passed, not during the event.

- Students may benefit from constructive creative outlets such as drama or arts to meet their expressive needs within the school day (e.g., in TJ's case, he found drawing to be helpful in expressing his feelings, and art classes were an appropriate outlet).

- Regular participation in strenuous, interest-based physical activity and involvement with positive peer groups such as sports teams may be useful to improve student's mood, stress levels, and social skills (e.g., in TJ's case, he experienced success with a recreational basketball league).

- Family interventions may also be recommended to assist the family in making environmental changes in the home (e.g., parents and caregivers may benefit from involvement in a parenting course, obtaining information from a child psychologist, and/or family counseling).

- A comprehensive assessment may reveal community-wide concerns (e.g., drug use, lack of recreational facilities, etc.) that inform the need for changes in the community.

Counseling Intervention

It is integral to a student's emotional well-being that a consistent and coordinated therapeutic approach be provided. The following interventions may be useful:

- Students may need individual counseling based on the need to address the following issues, as determined by their assessment results: attachment issues, family issues, and peer issues; suicidal ideation; addressing grief and abandonment issues as they arise; feelings of depression, anxiety, anger management; and stress management (e.g., in TJ's case, the development of a consistent therapeutic relationship was essential in addressing attachment and abandonment issues, as well as providing a safe place for TJ to explore his feelings of anger).

- Students with externalizing behaviors often require specific skills training in identifying and expressing emotions appropriately, instruction in self-calming techniques, and social skills training.

- Some students may struggle with talk therapy, and may benefit from more kinesthetic and creative treatments, such as clay work, play therapy, use of metaphors, narrative therapy, and/or art and drawing therapeutic strategies (e.g., TJ benefited from art therapy techniques, particularly drawing).

- Pro-social skills training in the community with a youth worker may help students develop their verbal and communication abilities.

- Self-esteem building through meaningful personal achievement via paid employment and/or volunteering in the community may be beneficial.

Educational/Vocational Planning

Students with externalizing behaviors may also present with educational difficulties (Ansary & Luthar, 2009). Depending on their strengths, their educational program may need to be modified to meet their specific needs. For example, TJ's present educational program continued to focus on "mainstream" academic success, as there were no reported difficulties with his cognitive functioning. However, due to TJ's strengths in physical performance, a hands-on, kinesthetic approach was of benefit when presenting new information and providing assigned tasks. Vocational goals were also modified to include his strengths in nonverbal reasoning, such as working with computers, electronics, and other devices. Other students may benefit from small group activities or modified class-work to address their academic concerns.

SUMMARY

A concise, complete, individualized intervention plan that targets the specific needs of the student can be developed using the results of a comprehensive as-sessment. In the case study in this chapter, a multi-disciplinary team was effective in thoroughly assessing the student's externalizing behaviors and developing in-sightful recommendations designed to move beyond controlling TJ's behaviors and providing support to TJ and those involved in his life.

Intervening with students who demonstrate externalizing behaviors requires a comprehensive assessment using standardized assessment instruments, risk assessment manuals, and, in some cases, targeted violence risk assessments (see Table 2.1). The case study of TJ illustrates how a professional school counselor, as part of a multi-disciplinary assessment team that also involves TJ's parents and caregivers, family physician, school administrators and teachers, as well as law en-forcement personnel, social workers and psychologists, can create an effective plan for intervention. Assessment via standardized assessments, the SAVRY, and a targeted violence risk assessment led to a comprehensive plan for reducing TJ's risk for violence and improve his functioning both at home and school. Successful use of comprehensive assessment tools can lead to well-planned, in-formed and defensible targeted plans for intervening with children who demon-strate externalizing behaviors.

REFERENCES

Achenbach, T. M., Krukowski, R. A., Dumenci, L., & Ivanova, M. Y. (2005). Assessment of adult psychopathology: Meta-analyses and implications of cross-informant correlations. *Psychological Bulletin, 131,* 361–382.

Achenbach, T. M., & Rescorla, L. A. (2001). *Manual for the ASEBA school-age forms & profiles.* Burlington, VT: University of Vermont, Research Center for Children, Youth, & Families, 2001.

American Psychiatric Association. (2000). *Diagnostic and statistical manual of mental disorders* (4th ed., Text Revision). Washington, DC: Author.

American School Counselor Association. (2004). *Ethical standards for school counselors.* Retrieved March 21, 2007, from http://www.schoolcounselor.org/files/ethical%20standards.pdf

Anderson-Butcher, D., Newsome, W. S., & Nay, S. (2003). Social skills intervention during elementary school recess: A visual analysis. *Children & Schools, 25,* 135–146.

Ansary, N. S., & Luthar, S. S. (2009). Distress and academic achievement among adolescents of affluence: A study of externalizing and internalizing problem behaviors and school performance. *Development and Psychopathology, 21*, 319–341.

Ash, P. (2002). Malpractice in child and adolescent psychiatry. *Child and Adolescent Psychiatric Clinics of North America, 11*, 869–885.

Astor, R. A., Benbenishty, R., & Meyer, H. A. (2004). Monitoring and mapping student victimization in schools. *Theory into Practice, 43*(1), 40–49.

Augimeri, L. K., Koegl, C. J., Webster, C. D., & Levene, K. (2001). *Early assessment risk list for boys, version 2.* Toronto, ON: Earlscourt Child and Family Center.

Beck, A. T., & Steer, R. A. (1993). *Beck hopelessness scale manual.* San Antonio, TX: The Psychological Corporation.

Beck, A. T., Steer, R. A., & Brown, G. K. (1996). *BDI–II manual.* San Antonio, TX: The Psychological Corporation.

Bernes, K. B., & Bardick, A. D. (2007). Conducting adolescent violence risk assessments: A framework for school counselors. *Professional School Counseling, 10*, 419–427.

Bongers, I. L., Koot, H. M., van der Ende, J., & Verhulst, F. C. (2004). Developmental trajectories of externalizing behaviors in childhood and adolescence. *Child Development, 75*, 1524–1537.

Borum, R., Bartel, F., & Forth, A. (2003). *Manual for the structured assessment of violence risk in youth.* Tampa, FL: University of South Florida.

Borum, R., & Reddy, M. (2001). Assessing violence risk in Tarasoff situations: A fact-based model of inquiry. *Behavioral Sciences and the Law, 19*, 375–385.

Cameron, J. K. (2000). Suicide threats in the aftermath of the Taber and Littleton shootings: How seriously do we take them? *The Canadian Psychological Association's Synopsis, 22*(4), 13.

Capuzzi, D. (2002). Legal and ethical challenges in counseling suicidal students. *Professional School Counseling, 6*, 36–35.

Conduct Problems Prevention Research Group. (1999). Initial impact of the Fast Track prevention trial for conduct problems: I. The high-risk sample. *Journal of Consulting and Clinical Psychology, 67*, 631–647.

Cormier, C. (1994). *Offender psycho-social assessment manual correctional model.* Penetanguishene, ON: Ontario Mental Health Centre.

Cornell, D. G., Sheras, P. L., Kaplan, S., McConville, D., Douglass, J., Elkon, A., McKnight, L., Branson, C., & Cole, J. (2004). Guidelines for student threat assessment: Field test findings. *School Psychology Review, 33*, 527–546.

Crothers, L. M., & Levinson, E. M. (2004). Assessment of bullying: A review of methods and instruments. *Journal of Counseling & Development, 82*, 496–503.

Cull, J. G., & Gill, W. S. (1988). *Suicide probability scale (SPS) manual.* Los Angeles, CA: Western Psychological Services.

Cullerton-Sen, C., & Crick, N. R. (2005). Understanding the effects of physical and relational victimization: The utility of multiple perspectives on predicting social-emotional adjustment. *School Psychology Review, 34*, 147–160.

Farrington, D. P. (2005). Understanding and preventing bullying. In M.Tonry (Ed.), *Crime and justice: A review of research* (pp. 381–458). Chicago: University of Chicago Press.

Frick, P. J. (2004). Developmental pathways to conduct disorder: Implications for serving youth who show severe aggressive and antisocial behavior. *Psychology in the Schools, 41*, 823–833.

Hernández, T. J., & Seem, S. R. (2004). A safe school climate: A systematic approach and the school counselor. *Professional School Counseling, 7*, 256–262.

Kauffman, J. M. (1999). How we prevent prevention of emotional and behavioral disorders. *Exceptional Children, 65*, 448–468.

Kovaks, M. (2001). *Children's depression inventory (CDI) manual.* North Tonawanda, NY: Multi-Health Systems.

Levene, K. S., Augimeri, L. K., Pepler, D. J., Walsh, M. M., Webster, C. D., & Koegl, C. J. (2001). *Early assessment risk list for girls, version 1, consultation edition.* Toronto, ON: Earlscourt Child and Family Center.

Lopes, J. A. (2007). Prevalence and comorbidity of emotional, behavioral and learning problems: a study of 7th-grade students. *Education & Treatment of Children, 30*, 165–181.

Liu, J. (2004). Childhood externalizing behaviors: Theory and implications. *Journal of Child and Adolescent Psychiatric Nursing, 17*, 93–103.

Merrill, K. M. (2008). *Behavioral, social, and emotional assessment of children and adolescents* (3rd ed.). New York: Lawrence Erlbaum.

Millon, T. (1993). *MACI manual: Millon adolescent clinical inventory.* Minneapolis, MN: NCS Pearson.

Mishna, F., & Alaggia, R. (2005). Weighing the risks: A child's decision to disclose peer victimization. *Children and Schools, 27*, 217–226.

Morgan, P. L., Farkas, G., & Wu, Q. (2009). Kindergarten predictors of recurring externalizing and internalizing psychopathology in the third and fifth grades. *Journal of Emotional and Behavioral Disorders, 17*, 67–79.

Niesyn, M. E. (2009). Strategies for success: Evidence-based instructional practices for students with emotional and behavioral disorders. *Preventing School Failure, 53*, 227–234.

Reynolds, C. R., & Kamphaus, R. W. (2004). *Behavior assessment system for children manual, second edition (BASC–2).* Circle Pines, MN: AGS Publishing.

Ross, D. M. (1996). *Childhood bullying and teasing: What school personnel, other professionals, and parents can do.* Alexandria, VA: American Counseling Association.

Singer, M., & Flannery, D. J. (2000). The relationship between children's threats of violence and violent behaviors. *Archives of Pediatric and Adolescent Medicine, 154*, 785–790.

Smith, D. C., & Sandhu, D. S. (2004). Toward a positive perspective on violence prevention in schools: Building connections. *Journal of Counseling & Development, 82*, 287–293.

Troop–Gordon, W., & Ladd, G. W. (2005). Trajectories of peer victimization and perceptions of the self and schoolmates: Precursors to internalizing and externalizing problems. *Child Development, 76*, 1072–1091.

Walker, B., Cheney, D., Stage, S., Blum, C., & Horner, R. H. (2005). Schoolwide screening and positive behavior supports. *Journal of Positive Behavior Interventions, 7*, 194–204.

Webster, C. D., Douglas, K. S., Eaves, D., & Hart, S. D. (1997). *HCR–20: Assessing risk for violence, Version 2.* Burnaby, BC: Mental Health, Law, and Policy Institute, Simon Fraser University.

Worthen, B. R., Borg, W. R., & White, K. R. (1993). *Measurement and evaluation in the schools: A practical guide.* White Plains, NY: Longman.

Chapter 3

Internalizing Behavior Disorders

Supporting Students with Depression, Anxiety, and Self-injurious Behavior

CHRISTOPHER A. SINK

Seattle Pacific University

Professional school counselors across grade levels support highly troubled students who are not necessarily showing behaviors reminiscent of an externalizing disorder (e.g., overt disruptive anti-social behavior, acting out). These students may exhibit indicators of even more self-destructive long-term mental health concerns, often referred to in the psychological/psychiatric literature as emotional or internalizing disorders (Colman, Wadsworth, Croudace, & Jones, 2007; Merrill, 2008; Morgan, Farkas, & Wu, 2009; Wolfe & Mash, 2006). What links, in part, the subject of this chapter to the subject of the previous chapter, externalizing behavior disorders, is persistent fear and anxiety, two major symptoms of internalizing disorders, which have also been associated with characteristics of externalizing disorders (Kramer & Zimmermann, 2009). This chapter first addresses how school counselors can better identify and assist K–12 students with potential depression and anxiety disorders, the most common internalizing disorders, although this category of disorders also includes such multifaceted and difficult to treat mental health issues such as bipolar disorders and post-traumatic stress disorder. Second, self-injurious behavior by the student is considered. This concern, as counselors can attest, presents major obstacles to address competently within school settings. For each of these mental health concerns, key research-based prevention and intervention approaches appropriate to school settings are discussed. Finally, resources for follow-up research are included as well.

ANXIETY AND DEPRESSION

School counselors must partner with other educators to help them recognize the warning signs of depression and anxiety. For instance, a student can be depressed and struggling with anxiety, but when a busy middle school science teacher with five large classes is asked about this teenager's recent behavior changes, the response might be, "Oh yeah, Jaime seems more quiet and preoccupied than usual. I just thought these ups and downs were fairly normal in early adolescents?"

As this teacher surmised, childhood depression and anxiety-related behaviors are frequently not severe enough to warrant medical classification or labeling. Normally, the symptoms are relatively short-lived and dissipate without intense psychotherapy or medical intervention. In such cases, school counselors can lend their support to students and their parents, caregivers, and teachers. However, if untreated, clinical levels of depression and anxiety can have harmful long-term educational, psychosocial, and physical consequences (Colman et al., 2007). These students can also develop eating disorders, school and/or social phobias, cutting behavior, and suicidal ideations. At this level of severity, a mental health professional should already be assisting the student. The goal for professional school counselors, of course, is to intervene prior to the problems becoming full disorders.

Before reviewing the primary signs of depression and anxiety, the following real-world case study is provided. The student, Amy, shows signs of developing an internalizing or mood disorder, a subcategory of the National Institute of Mental Health's (NIMH; 2009) classification system. Consider these questions while reading the scenario: Is she depressed, anxious, or both? How might a school counselor attend to her needs?

After reading about Amy's situation, one observes that she is not only experiencing depression, but it is coupled with significant worries. In fact, certain children and youth experience symptoms of depression and anxiety more or less independently of each other. Some, like Amy, report feeling both emotions concurrently (Anderson & Hope, 2008; Doll & Cummings, 2008; Kessler, Berglund, Demler, Jin, & Walters, 2005; Sink & Igelman, 2004). Whether the school counselor should refer a student like Amy to an outside mental health professional for an evaluation and possible intervention, while continuing to support her in the school setting, is influenced by several factors (e.g., student's familial

Amy: A School-Based Case Study[1]

Amy, a 15-year-old high school sophomore, is self-referred to the school counselor. As Amy walks into the school counselor's office, her facial expression is blank, except for a slight frown. She slumps down in the chair across from the counselor without saying a word. She is dressed in baggy, oversized jeans, a black-hooded sweatshirt, and several long medallion-style necklaces. After several attempts to make eye contact with Amy, the counselor prompts her for an explanation as to why she referred herself, and Amy begins to speak in a quiet tone and at a slow pace. She explains that she believes she is suffering from depression and is hoping for some assistance in finding free on-going counseling services and a prescription for medication. Both of these, she states, are in an effort to relieve her depressive symptoms.

The school counselor begins to ask Amy a few questions about her life at home and learns the following: Amy has spent the past two years living in a section of town that might be classified as lower-middle class, in an older two-bedroom, one-story home. She has been raised solely by her mother, who works every day at an office building in town and spends most nights continuing to work from home. Though Amy is unsure of her mother's exact title, she understands that it has something to do with the real estate business. When her mother is not working, she apparently fills her free time with a boyfriend, who spends the night in the home on a fairly regular basis. Amy expresses great concern and frustration over her mother's choice of companion, and mentions that she tries to spend as much time away from the home as possible. She admits that she worries a lot about her mother's happiness but has an extremely difficult time communicating with her mother about anything and believes that even if she tried, her mother would never understand where she's coming from. Perhaps even more importantly, Amy believes her mother does not understand her at all, especially the fact that Amy chooses to spend so much time away from home.

This is Amy's first year at this high school, and it is her second year living in the city. She has found a small group of other students with whom she is friendly, but she admits that there is only one friend, Keisha, with whom she socializes with outside of school. When Amy is not spending time with Keisha, she says that she prefers to be volunteering at the local animal shelter, taking care of and playing with the animals. Her career goal is to be involved in a project to save certain breeds of dogs from poor treatment in Alaska. Part of her interest in animals, Amy explains, stems from the fact that she rarely feels understood by people (family, friends, etc.), and appreciates the unconditional love she receives from the animals. Apart from animals, Amy's second largest interest is in anime (Japanese animation) and Japanese culture.

The school counselor then questions Amy about her schoolwork and learns that the Amy believes she is not being challenged in any of her classes. Amy admits she usually understands everything that is going on during lessons, but due to her disinterest in the material she fails to turn in most of the assignments, and seems not to care about her school performance. As a result, Amy's grades are dropping rapidly. Last year in middle school, Amy was getting mostly As and Bs. In contrast, her current grades are Cs and Ds.

Amy has recently learned that she will be moving to another city in a couple of months. She is glad to be moving away from a place where she has never felt understood and hates most of the students and teachers at the school. On the other hand, she mentions that she is worried about the transition to a new school and her ability to again start the process of meeting new friends and finding her niche.

---

1. This student's story was provided by a high school counselor, Ms. Jenna Shallenberger, in the Puget Sound area of Washington state. This is not the student's actual name.

context, the severity of her symptoms, and the impact on her education). In any case, school counselors must initially ask themselves: Do the student's emotional and social challenges fit the well-documented pattern of major childhood depression and anxiety? A review of the essential characteristics and the epidemiology of depression and anxiety can help school counselors answer this question and plan effective school-based intervention strategies.

CHARACTERISTICS OF DEPRESSION AND ANXIETY DISORDERS

Before discussing serious student depression and anxiety problems that are diagnosable by highly trained mental health professionals, the common warning signs of *early-onset* depression and anxiety are summarized below. Obviously, as the signs become more intense, longer-lasting, and frequent, the greater the probability that the indicators point to a depressive or anxiety disorder (Merrill, 2008).

Depression—Early Warning Signs

Ranging from mild to severe, symptoms of depression in children and youth can also be accompanied by anxiety-related behaviors. Here are key early warning signs of emerging depression:

- Persistent sadness and hopelessness (over at least one full year for children and youth)
- Lack of enthusiasm, energy, or motivation
- Increased irritability or agitation
- Withdrawal from friends and from activities the student once enjoyed
- Changes in eating and sleeping habits
- Indecision, lack of concentration, or forgetfulness
- Missing school or poor school performance
- Poor self-esteem, shame, or guilt
- Significant problems with parents and caregivers
- Frequent physical complaints, such as headaches and stomachaches
- Drug and/or alcohol use and abuse
- Self mutilation
- Thoughts of death and/or suicidal ideations (Horowitz & Garber, 2006; National Alliance on Mental Illness, 2009, n.p.)

Untreated depressive symptoms will eventually detract from healthy development and negatively impact daily life. For instance, elementary-age students with depression may, by early adolescence, develop additional personal (e.g., anxiety, eating, substance abuse, or externalizing disorders) and educational challenges (e.g., receiving a higher proportion of suspensions or expulsions, school failure; Gillham, Shatte, & Freres, 2000; Rudolph, Hammen, & Daley, 2006) that will require focused intervention.

Anxiety—Early Warning Signs

Students with nascent anxiety or anxiety disorders experience the interrelated feelings of substantial fear, worry, and/or nervousness associated with emotional pain and/or avoidance reactions (Kendall, Hedtke, & Aschenbrand, 2006). Emotions such as these can last for months, even years, and, if intense enough, will noticeably alter the student's day-to-day functioning. Accordingly, if the anxiety symptoms are not attended to early on, students can develop any number of these additional challenges:

- Recurring school problems (e.g., missing school, low grades)
- Interpersonal difficulties, especially with peers
- Low self-worth and a sad affect
- Physical health challenges
- Substance abuse
- Problems with work-related adjustment
- Anxiety disorder (e.g., Kendall et al., 2006; Murray, Creswell, & Cooper, 2009; Substance Abuse and Mental Health Services Administration's [SAMHSA] National Mental Health Information Center, 2003)

FROM EARLY WARNING SIGNS TO DEPRESSION AND ANXIETY DISORDERS

As with any serious, ongoing emotional challenge, early warning signs can evolve into a clinically identifiable disorder. Students with depressive or anxiety disorders will present a constellation of emotional and behavioral symptoms. The etiologies of each disorder vary widely, including genetic, biochemical, familial, and psychosocial explanations. Generally speaking, however, professional school counselors will find that students with depressive disorders frequently experience some overlapping with symptoms of anxiety disorders (Flannery-Schroeder, 2006), such as nervousness, touchiness, sleep problems, and difficulty concentrating. Because of this pattern, it is not a simple matter to differentiate those who are showing signs of an emerging depressive or anxiety disorder (Anderson & Hope, 2008; Kendall et al., 2006; Merrill, 2008; Rudolph et al., 2006).

Identifying and labeling mental disorders are complicated by the fact that the medical model, with its non-educational terminology, is the dominant classification paradigm used by mental health professionals. Although it is beyond this chapter's scope to discuss at length the American Psychiatric Association's (2000) *Diagnostic and Statistical Manual of Mental Disorders, Text Revision* (DSM–IV–TR), the publication includes three relevant sections that are associated with school-age internalizing disorders: (1) Disorders Usually First Diagnosed in Infancy, Childhood, or Adolescence[2]; (2) Anxiety Disorders (e.g., panic disorder, social phobia, obsessive-compulsive disorder [OCD], post-traumatic stress disorder [PTSD]); and, (3) Mood Disorders (e.g., depressive and bipolar disorders). The subtypes related to anxiety and mood disorders are multifaceted and require significant DSM–IV–TR training to decipher. As a quick reference, they are summarized in Table 3.1. For detailed information on the disorders and their subtypes[3], the manual is a good place to start.

Age of Onset and Prevalence Rates

The age of onset of diagnosable depression and anxiety is not thoroughly documented for the current generation of school-age children and youth. Subtypes of depression or anxiety disorders will vary in when specific symptoms appear during childhood or adolescence (Kendall et al., 2006; Roza, Hofstra, van der Ende, & Verhulst, 2003; Rudolph et al., 2006). It is important to note that adults with persistent depression often report that their depressive episodes began during adolescence (Avenevoli, Knight, Kessler, & Merikangas, 2008; Cuijpers, Straten, Smits, & Smit, 2006).

Statistics about the overall mental health of school-age children are widely available. For example, the Surgeon General's (U.S. Department of Health and Human Services, 1999) mental health report estimated that approximately 5% to 9% of children and adolescents ages 9 to 17 in the United States have an emotional disturbance (ED). The Surgeon General further estimated that 3.5 million severely disturbed children are not receiving any substantial intervention (U.S. Public Health Service, 2000). It is also estimated that about 4.3 million American youth who experience mental disorders tend to have significant problems at home and school, as well as in peer relationships (InCrisis, 2007).

A national survey of parents and caregivers revealed that the mean percentage of children ages 4–17 in the United States with significant emotional and behavioral difficulties was about 5% (2006 data cited from Forum on Child and Family Statistics, 2008). For the same age range, disaggregated by gender, the mean percentages were approximately 7% for boys and 3% for girls. Lower socio-economic status (SES) also seems to be linked with increased emotional and behavioral difficulties. On average about 8.5% of the children living below

---

[2]This section includes no depressive disorders and only one anxiety disorder—that is, separation anxiety disorder (SAD; DSM-IV-TR diagnostic criteria 309.21). SAD is characterized by a disproportionate (developmentally inappropriate) level of anxiety (lasting at least 4 weeks) when away from their home or from their significant others to whom they are emotionally attached. To be diagnosed with SAD, children under 18, must display clinically significant symptoms (e.g., repeated separation-themed nightmares, complaints of somatic problems like head and stomach aches, and persistent worrying about losing a loved and refusal of attending school) which negatively influence social, academic (occupational), and/or other areas of functioning.

[3]Note. K-12 students who exhibit characteristics of other anxiety or depressive disorders are classified according to DSM-IV-TR using the criteria enumerated under either the Anxiety Disorders or Mood Disorders sections (see Table 3.1).

T A B L E 3.1   **Summary of Mood Disorders and Anxiety Disorders from DSM–IV–TR (American Psychiatric Association, 2000)**

Diagnostic Type & Subtypes		Code	Essential Features	Age of Onset
			Mood Disorders	
Depressive Disorders	Major Depressive Disorder — Single event	296.2x	Symptoms of severe depression which arise for the initial time	Any age; average onset age = mid-20s
	Re-current	296.3x	Two or more major depressive events with an intervening time interval of 2 consecutive months.	
	Dysthymic Disorder	300.4	Chronic depression for most of the day lasting at least for a 1-year-period.	Any age; early onset < age 21
			Premenstrual dysphoric disorder (PDD; must be severe enough to interfere with school/work);	
	Depression Disorder Not otherwise specified (NOS)	311	*Minor depressive disorder* (MDD; at least 2 but < 5 depressive episodes) with symptoms (e.g., for children and youth irritable and/or depressed mood, lack of interest/pleasure in most activities, sleep and weight issues, low self worth);	Early onset < age 21
			Recurrent brief depressive disorder (depressive episodes lasting from 2 days to < 2 weeks, occurring ≥ once a month for 1 year) with symptoms (identical to Major Depressive Episodes but lasting < 2 weeks).	
Bipolar Disorders	Bipolar I Disorder with six expressions	296.0x – 296.7	Depression coupled with manic symptoms (specifics for each subtype are available in DSM–IV–TR)	Occurs in school-age children; mean onset age = 20

(*Continued*)

T A B L E 3.1 Summary of Mood Disorders and Anxiety Disorders from DSM-IV-TR (American Psychiatric Association, 2000) (Continued)

Diagnostic Type & Subtypes		Code	Essential Features	Age of Onset
Mood Disorders				
Bipolar II Disorder (Hypomanic-Depressed)		296.89	More than one Major Depressive Episode and at least one Hypomanic Episode (i.e., persistent and pervasive elated or irritable mood, and behaviors and thoughts)	Occurs in school-age children
Cyclothymic Disorder		301.13	Frequent periods with (and without) symptoms for no less than 2 months at a time) hypomanic and depressive symptoms enduring for at least 1 year.	Typical onset in adolescence or early adulthood
Bipolar Disorder (NOS)		296.80	Disorders with bipolar attributes that do not meet diagnostic criteria for any specific Bipolar Disorder	Not stated
Mood Disorder Due to a Medical Condition		293.83	Due to a general medical/physiological condition or physiological effects of a substance (e.g., illegal drug, prescribed medication), individuals experience a major and persistent disturbance in mood that pervades their clinical situation; a depressed mood and/or an elevated, expansive, or irritable mood.	Not stated
Mood Disorder Due Substance-Induced Disorder				
Mood Disorder NOS		296.90	Mood symptoms that do not meet the criteria for any specific Mood Disorder.	Not stated
Anxiety Disorders				
Panic Disorder	With Agora-phobia	300.01	An unexpected onset of intense nervousness, fear, or terror which can include agoraphobia (anxiety about, or evasion of, circumstances from which escape would be challenging or embarrassing), including such symptoms as shortness of breath, palpitations and discomfort in chest, fear of "going crazy"	Late adolescence to mid-30s
	No Agora-phobia	300.21		

Disorder	Code	Description	Onset
Agoraphobia Without History of Panic Disorder	300.22	Anxiety about, or evasion of, circumstances from which escape would be challenging or embarrassing.	Undetermined
Specific Phobia	300.29	Clinically significant anxiety caused by contact with a particular feared thing or situation. Avoidance of that object or situation often follows.	Usually in childhood or early teens
Social Phobia	300.23	Clinically significant anxiety caused by contact with a particular social or performance situations. Avoidance of that object or situation often follows.	Typically mid-adolescence, but at times early childhood
Obsessive-Compulsive Disorder (OCD)	300.3	Obsessive behavior that generates significant anxiety and distress and/or compulsions which seem to ameliorate the anxiety	Normally in adolescence, but also in childhood
Posttraumatic Stress Disorder (PTSD)	309.81	Re-experiencing of a highly traumatic situation that leads to heightened stimulation and avoidance behavior (symptoms arise within 3 months of trauma)	Occurs at any age, including childhood
Acute Stress Disorder	308.3	Symptoms of PTSD immediately following an exceedingly distressing incident.	Not specified
Generalized Anxiety Disorder (GAD)	300.02	Constant anxiety for at least 6 months	Onset can occur in childhood or adolescence
Anxiety Disorder Due to General Medical Condition	293.84	Serious anxiety as a result of some physiological cause.	Not specified
Substance-Induced Anxiety Disorder		Major anxiety induced by a substance (illegal or legal medication, toxin exposure)	
Anxiety Disorder NOS	300.00	Disorders with prominent anxiety or phobic avoidance that do not meet the criteria for any specific Anxiety Disorder, Adjustment Disorder with Anxiety, or Adjustment Disorder with Mixed Anxiety and Depressed Mood.	Not specified

NOTE: Roughly speaking, to be classified as "disordered", students should exhibit symptoms that are severe enough to generally lead to significant personal-social distress and impairments to their daily functioning at school, home, work, etc.

100% poverty are reported to exhibit these concerns. Children living in families with fewer than two caregivers have a somewhat higher risk of developing emotional and behavioral problems. According to a 2001 study, the prevalence of emotional, behavioral, and developmental problems was the highest among children living in poverty (5.5%), among adolescents ages 12 to 17 (5.0%), and among boys (4.7%; Centers for Disease Control and Prevention, 2005).

In summary, for both girls and boys, the conservative prevalence rate for childhood and adolescent depression is around 5% (American Academy of Child & Adolescent Psychiatry, 2008). For school-age students, up to perhaps 13% are experiencing significant anxiety. Children living at the lower end of the socio-economic spectrum and girls appear to experience higher rates of anxiety and depression, but boys are more likely to be diagnosed with an emotional disability than girls. Though not discussed here, the prevalence rates for particular subtypes of depression and anxiety disorders are available in the DSM–IV–TR and in more technical books (e.g., Kendall et al., 2006; Rudolph et al., 2006). Finally, although roughly 5% of K–12 students have an emotional disturbance, only 1% of those receive treatment (Reddy & Richardson, 2006). Thus, there is a substantial need for effective school-based screening, prevention, and intervention services.

ANXIETY AND DEPRESSION DISORDERS IN SPECIAL EDUCATION LANGUAGE

The label "emotional disturbance" (ED) is used in Public Law 108–446 or the Individuals with Disabilities Act (IDEA; U.S. Department of Education, 2004, 2009) when referring to elementary- to secondary-age students with a diagnosable but unspecified emotional, behavioral, or mental disorder that severely limits their functioning in various developmental domains (e.g., social, academic, and emotional). Two of the five ED characteristics include chronic symptoms related to students with severe depression (i.e., an all-encompassing disposition of unhappiness or depression) and major anxiety (i.e., propensity to develop physical symptoms or fears related to personal or school difficulties; National Dissemination Center for Children with Disabilities publication [NICHCY], 2004). Those students who have been diagnosed with a depressive or anxiety disorder then may be assigned the ED designation and receive appropriate special education services. Less than 25% of students identified as ED show the expressions of an internalizing disorder (Dwyer, 2002). It is also common to hear educators and parent advocacy groups using the label "emotional and behavior disorder" (EBD) in reference to students with an ED. Finally, students with mild forms of anxiety and/or depression may receive a "504 plan" (see Section 504 of the Rehabilitation Act; U.S. Department of Education, 2009) to help them in the short-term with their adjustment issues. In the next section, best-practice recommendations are discussed to assist students with depression and anxiety.

RECOMMENDATIONS FOR SCHOOL
COUNSELING PRACTICE

Professional school counselors are vital members of students' support systems. Below are realistic, research-based ideas that begin at the broad programmatic level and progress to more specific suggestions.

Implement a Comprehensive School Counseling Program

First, as part of a recommended ecological approach to working with a student's anxiety and depression (Abrams, Theberge, & Karan, 2005), make sure the school's or school district's comprehensive school counseling program (CSCP; e.g., American School Counselor Association's [2005] National Model; Dollarhide & Saginak, 2008; Gysbers & Henderson, 2006) includes an effective K–12 responsive services module. Such a module should be evidence-based and incorporate effective screening processes for mental health problems (e.g., internalizing and externalizing disorders) as well as proven school-based prevention and intervention strategies. Moreover, given that students' mental health is influenced by various intrinsic and extrinsic psychosocial protective dimensions and vulnerability factors (Walsh, 2006), K–12 school counselors, under the aegis of a comprehensive school counseling program, need to create a nurturing and supportive learning environment (Sink & Edwards, 2008; Slater & McKeown, 2004). The steps that follow expand, in part, on these overall recommendations.

Create and Implement a System of Positive
Behavior Support (PBS)

According to IDEA, school districts must use research-based positive behavioral supports and systematic and individual interventions when addressing the social-emotional needs of children and youth with disabilities (Dunlap, Carr, Horner, Zarcone, & Schwartz, 2008; Handler, Rey, Connell, Thier, Feinberg, & Putnam, 2007). These are often specified in their individual educational programs. Because a positive behavior support system is designed to be preventative and proactive through collaborative, data-based decision-making (Safrin, 2006) and implemented school-wide (see Doll & Cummings, 2008, for several examples) it can be readily aligned with the responsive services component of CSCPs (Gysbers & Henderson, 2006). Rather than focusing on negative and retaliatory methods of school and classroom management, positive behavior support procedures and processes attempt to not only reduce the occurrence of challenging behaviors and emotions exhibited by students with disorders, but also to enhance their prosocial skill set (Carr, 2007). Strategies to accomplish this objective may include school counselors in the following ways:

- Working with a positive behavior support team of relevant educators (e.g., a school psychologist, regular and special educators, a school administrator) to develop and implement proactive and positive school-wide behavior management plan

- Co-leading a social skills curriculum with classroom teachers
- Assisting teachers in making appropriate learning accommodations
- Providing parent/caregiver education
- Conducting individual and small group interventions founded on functional behavioral assessments (Bambara & Kern, 2005; Galassi & Akos, 2007; Sink & Edwards, 2008).

These activities should be implemented in conjunction with the next recommendation.

Establish and Implement Prevention Activities in Conjunction with a School-Based Mental Health Screening Plan

The first line of defense for the successful prevention of and intervention in student depression and anxiety is an effective mental health screening process (Weist, Rubin, Moore, Adelsheim, & Wrobel, 2007).

K–12 school counselors can partner with their school psychologist and other mental health professionals to establish the screening procedures and processes. A recent meta-analysis showed that school-based interventions implemented after screening students for depression are more successful than those without such a screening process in place (Cuijpers et al., 2006). At the very least, school counselors can help facilitate a multi-disciplinary team or student assistance team that regularly meets to screen and assist students with significant challenges affecting their educational, emotional, and behavioral functioning. Team members should include the school nurse, school psychologist, relevant teachers, and the school administrator. New Mexico has an excellent example of a Student Assistance Team Manual available for download at http://www.ped.state.nm.us/resources/downloads/dl/file.2.pdf.

Elementary school counselors will want to review the literature for research-based screening programs, familiarizing themselves especially with the very widely used Systematic Screening for Behavior Disorders process (SSBD; Walker, Severson, Nicholson, Kehle, Jenson, & Clark, 1994; see also Merchant, Anderson, Caldarella, Fisher, Young, & Young, 2009) used with K–6 students at risk for developing either an externalizing or internalizing behavior disorder. Another excellent resource to consult for screening instruments is Reddy and Richardson's (2006) publication. It summarizes such well-researched elementary school screening and intervention programs as *First Step to Success* and *Parent-Teacher Action Research* (PTAR). Using *First Step*'s coherent and standardized process, kindergartners exhibiting early signs of internalizing and externalizing behavior disorders are proactively screened by their classroom teachers. Once the high-risk students are identified, they are further assessed with various formal screening measures as well as observed systematically in classrooms. As needed, effective whole-school prevention and intervention methods (see Reddy, Newman, De Courtney, & Chun,

2009) are later initiated and supported by relevant educators such as school counselors. On a case-by-case basis, outside mental health professionals may also assist the school. Similar processes and procedures are implemented with PTAR, but parents and caregivers are more actively involved in the screening-prevention-intervention sequence.

Because students in later grades will need to be identified as well, quality screening processes must be in place. Again, school counselors, school psychologists, and special educators can help organize, implement, and evaluate this critical service. Good assessment resources are readily available for addressing emotional problems in general (Erford, 2007), and anxiety disorders (Kendall et al., 2006) and depressive disorders (Rudolph et al., 2006) in particular.

Work Toward Prevention

School-based prevention strategies and activities should be instituted at all grade levels (Barrett & Pahl, 2006; Horowitz & Garber, 2006), with special emphasis placed on the elementary grades. Sample prevention programs and activities available to elementary school counselors are outlined in Reddy and Richardson (2006) and elsewhere (e.g., Martinez & Nellis, 2008; Poulou, 2005). These largely focus on teaching effective coping and social skills to students and providing both parent/caregiver and regular education teacher assistance to children who are showing early signs of depression and anxiety. The more knowledgeable teachers and caregivers are about depression signs and symptoms, the better the chance of appropriate, early referrals to school counselors (Auger, 2005). School counselors can offer training to teachers as ongoing quarterly in-services and during regular staff meetings (Abrams et al., 2005; Auger). Parent in-services can be held in the evenings so working parents can attend.

Effective prevention also includes school counselors helping students reach positive developmental competencies (see, e.g., American School Counselor Association's [2005] national model's personal-social competencies) and equipping them with the cognitive-socio-emotional skills (e.g., recognition, identification, and expression of emotions; self-awareness, and impulsivity control; teamwork, empathy, caring about oneself and others) to successfully adapt to the stressful circumstances in their daily lives (Poulou, 2005). Moreover, in order to assist students in recognizing and taking positive steps toward healthy living, school counselors need to be promoting overall wellness and healthy emotional development (Martinez & Nellis, 2008; see Poulou for a review of multiple programs).

Regrettably, effective school-based approaches targeted specifically to prevent and support students experiencing depression and anxiety are not well documented in the literature (Gillham et al. 2007; Masia-Warner, Nangle, & Hansen, 2006). There is some research support, however, for conducting small group activities and classroom guidance lessons that teach coping strategies to students at risk for emotional problems.

Establish and Implement Intervention Services   After screening procedures and classroom guidance have been implemented as systemic-ecological prevention tools (Abrams et al., 2005), those students with more severe emotional challenges, such as depression and anxiety, will almost certainly require additional research-based and school counseling-related services, including peer support groups, small group work, and individual counseling. Although beyond the scope of this chapter, one promising school-based "systems" model, Response to Intervention (RTI), is gaining traction in the professional literature (see Martinez & Nellis, 2008, for an overview). Like so many new approaches, RTI's efficacy for school counseling applications has yet to be validated.

Peer Support   While the usefulness of peer support or peer helping groups with students with emotional concerns has yet to be established, a number of education and school counseling-related publications suggest that these type of groups can be somewhat effective (e.g., Baginsky, 2004; Burns & Hulusi, 2005; Drop & Block, 2004; Lewis & Lewis, 1996; Oswald & Mazefskey, 2006; Slater & McKeown, 2004; Tobias, 2001). It may therefore be a good idea to pilot a peer support group and monitor its helpfulness to students with emotional problems.

Small Group Counseling   Following the implementation of large group guidance activities and peer helping programs, small group counseling is the next intervention level school counselors should try. Multiple articles published over the past decade in the *Journal for Specialists in Group Work* and elsewhere (e.g., in *Professional School Counseling*) provide ample information on this service. For example, school counselors may want to run psychoeducational and rational emotive behavioral counseling groups for students with depression and anxiety (see Auger, 2005; Sommers-Flanagan, Barrett-Hakanson, Clarke, & Sommers-Flanagan, 2000). Specific research-based goals for group counseling interventions should center on increasing students' (A) awareness of their emotions and those of others, (B) peer support system, (C) use of appropriate social skills through role-playing and other means, (D) self-care (e.g., scheduling enjoyable and rewarding activities), and (E) personal strengths (Auger; McWhirter & Burrow, 2001). Sample catalyzing activities summarized in Auger might include using emotional vocabulary cards, where developmentally appropriate feeling words are written on index cards, and then students draw cards one by one and explain a situation in their lives where they experienced this emotion. Another helpful activity to help students gauge their emotional health and make connections between the influence of emotions in different situations involves the school counselor drawing a large emotional thermometer and having students provide examples of situations and the feelings associated with them. Students can point to the thermometer to indicate the strength of the experienced emotions, placing them on a continuous scale of intensity from least to most intense as the "temperature" of the emotions increases. Finally, rational emotive behavior counseling groups with specific grade-level interventions have been found to be useful (McWhirter & Burrow). Again, in these groups, principal topics to consider are: feelings, behavior, self-acceptance, decision-making, and so on.

Referral and Supportive Individual Counseling   Students exhibiting signs of depression and anxiety often require a referral to outside mental health professionals. The research indicates that cognitive-behavioral therapy (CBT) has been found to be more effective than behavioral or cognitive therapy alone (see reviews in Auger, 2005; McWhirter & Burrow, 2001; Oswald & Mazefskey, 2006; Sink & Igelman, 2004; Weisz, McCarty, & Valeri, 2006). Because cognitive behavioral therapy and behavioral interventions are intensive counseling modalities and can be long-term, school counselors need to assist families in locating therapists who are properly trained in these methods as well as knowledgeable of medications. It must be noted, however, that the psychotherapeutic methods sometimes used to treat internalizing disorders require further research to confirm their efficacy with children and youth (Oswald & Mazefskey).

Whether students with depression or anxiety are receiving outside counseling or not, school counselors, using a strengths-based approach (Galassi & Akos, 2007), should continue to support these students and their families. Seeing students on an individual basis can be very helpful. Obviously, for individual supportive counseling to be more useful, school counselors need to be particularly caring and empathic with the students experiencing emotional challenges (Auger, 2005). Individual sessions should assist students to understand and experience the connections among thoughts, feelings, and actions; set realistic goals and monitor progress toward the goals; identify their developmental assets and reframe their self defeating belief patterns (i.e., negative, unproductive, unrealistic beliefs about self, others, and their circumstances); recognize and change their self destructive behaviors; better cope with stressful situations; and enhance their enjoyment of regular daily activities (Curry & Reinecke, 2003; Galassi & Akos; McWhirter & Burrow, 2001). Finally, research suggests that increased physical activity is associated with a lessening of depressive symptoms (Auger). As such, school counselors can partner with physical education teachers and coaches to create an individualized fitness plans for their students.

Working with a School Nurse on Medication Issues   When students with depression and anxiety are prescribed psychotropic medications to supplement behavioral and psychosocial interventions, school counselors, with assistance from the family and the school nurse, should ethically consult with the student's physicians (e.g., pediatrician, child psychiatrist). It is not critical to know all the available drugs and their side effects because these facts are regularly updated at the *Physician's Desk Reference* Web site (http://www.pdrhealth.com/). However, to further support students, families, and teachers, school counselors should have some familiarity with the classes of medications used specifically to treat childhood anxiety and depression and how these drugs might affect the student's learning and school behavior (see Abrams, Flood, & Phelps, 2006, for details). Frequently prescribed medications for anxiety and/or depression-related symptoms are presented in Table 3.2. Abrams et al. lists the major side effects of these medications that may negatively impact school learning, including drowsiness and fatigue, other physical symptoms (e.g., dizziness, headaches, dry mouth, restlessness, decreased appetite, nausea), and potential cognitive impairment. Of course, not all medications will

T A B L E   3.2   Common Psychotropic Medications Administered to Children and Youth with Depression and Anxiety (Abrams et al., 2006)

Medication Name (Trade Name)	Used to Treat
Buspirone (BuSpar)	Generalized anxiety disorder (GAD), social phobia
Clomipramine (Anafranil)	Obsessive compulsive disorder (OCD), depression
Clonazepam (Klonopin)	GAD, separation anxiety, panic attacks
Clonidine (Catapres)	Post-traumatic stress disorder (PTSD)
Fluoxetine (Prozac)	OCD, social phobia, depression
Fluvoxamine (Luvox)	Depression, GAD, OCD, social phobia, separation anxiety
Nefazodone (Serzone)	Depression
Paroxetine (Paxil)	Adolescent depression, OCD
Propranolol (Inderal)	PTSD
Sertraline (Zoloft)	OCD, depression

produce all of these side effects. Other side effects not listed may occur. Moreover, the side effects may vary in intensity, frequency, and duration. It is common, however, that the side effects are the strongest during the first few weeks or even months after first starting on the medications. During this initial period when the medications are beginning to take effect, school counselors should work closely with the student's family, physician, teachers, school psychologist, and the school nurse, making sure the child's education does not suffer too much.

SELF-INJURIOUS BEHAVIOR (SIB)

Regrettably, this teen's story is not an isolated occurrence. Similar cases are found throughout the psychological and educational literature (Lloyd-Richardson, Nock, & Prinstein, 2009). One relevant study surveyed elementary and secondary school counselors drawn from a large American School Counselor Association database (Roberts-Dobie & Donatelle, 2007). Over three-fourths ($N = 518$, 81%) of

---

Cleo: A School-Based Case Study

Hemorrhaging slightly from her wrist area, Cleo, a high school junior, was found by a friend in a bathroom stall digging at her skin with a ball-point pen. When confronted by her friend, Cleo grimacing with pain, nervously covered up her arm and indicated that she was just "making a cool tattoo". The friend had the good sense to immediately report the event and conversation to her school counselor, who then followed up with Cleo and her family. Appropriate referrals were made as well.

the sample reported working with a self-injurer at least once during their career. Thus, reminiscent of the other mental health issues discussed in this chapter and book, school counselors have an important role in assisting students who may be at-risk for self-injurious behavior (SIB) and with those already receiving treatment from outside clinicians. The essential elements of SIB and school-based activities to support students and their families are summarized below.

Characteristics and Prevalence Rates

Teenagers with psychological issues such as depression and anxiety may also engage in the self-infliction of pain. Although there are subtle differences in terminology (i.e., deliberate self-harming [DSH], self-destructive, self-injurious, self-mutilating behavior), researchers are largely describing an analogous phenomenon. *Self-injurious behavior* (SIB), with its suicidal (SSI) and nonsuicidal (NSSI) dimensions, is generally seen as an umbrella term (Prinstein, 2008). Along with numerous useful publications and web sites on this subject (e.g., Klonsky, 2007; Kress, Gibson, Reynolds, 2004; Laye-Gindhu & Schonert-Reichl, 2005; Nixon & Heath, 2009; Nock, Joiner, Gordon, Lloyd-Richardson, & Prinstein, 2006; Roberts-Dobie & Donatelle, 2007; YouthNet UK, 2009), Cornell University's (n.d.) Research Program on Self-Injurious Behavior in Adolescents and Young Adults provides a wealth of information to consult.

Even though the most familiar method of self-injury among adolescents and young adults is deliberate cutting (Craigen & Foster, 2009; Roberts-Dobie & Donatelle, 2007), there are other disturbing manifestations, including head-banging and hitting other body parts against hard surfaces, biting, breaking bones, burning and scalding, hair pulling, jumping from heights or in front of vehicles, excessive scratching of the skin, stabbing, and/or swallowing objects or inserting objects into the body. Minimal body-piercing (e.g., earrings or eyebrow posts) as a way of expressing oneself culturally should not initially be associated with chronic self-injurious behavior. As alluded to above, students with SIB occasionally entertain suicidal ideations and in some cases may act on them (Craigen & Foster; Prinstein, 2008). Further complicating the issue, adolescent SIB has been linked to other serious mental health concerns including eating disorders (Levitt, Sansone, & Cohn, 2004; Ross, Heath, & Toste, 2009), substance abuse, and Borderline Personality Disorder (BPD; Sansone & Levitt, 2005; see APA's [2000] *Diagnostic and Statistical Manual of Mental Disorders IV–TR* for additional information), but the extent and nature of this relationship are not well understood. For these reasons alone SIB can be a very dangerous psychological condition that requires immediate professional mental health and perhaps medical consultation and intervention.

NSSI Causes and Correlates   Although epidemiological studies report varying prevalence rates (see Heath, Schaub, Holly, & Nixon, 2009; Nock & Prinstein, 2005; Prinstein, 2008; Rodham & Hawton, 2009, for summaries), there is consensus that NSSI generally has an early-to-late adolescence onset (Lloyd-Richardson et al., 2009). One to 4% of the general population has been diagnosed as NSSI. However, depending on the study, this rate increases considerably among nonclinical (community) samples of preteens (7%) and adolescents (14% to 39%), as well as among adolescents (21% to 61%) in clinical samples. Other researchers suggest that about 15% to 20% of adolescents in the community disclose they have engaged in NSSI at least once (Heath et al.). NSSI tends to occur more often in females, but prevalence rates among other demographic subgroups (e.g., by ethnicity and socio-economic status) are unknown. Regrettably, the studies investigating SIB's potential risk factors are inconclusive (Prinstein). They appear to be numerous, interdependent, and complicated to untangle (Klonsky & Glenn, 2009).

Moreover, the reasons for NSSI and what precipitates the behavior are not well understood. Researchers suggest that familial, sociological, psychological, and neurobiological factors contribute to the onset of NSSI (Lloyd-Richardson et al., 2009; Osuch & Payne, 2009). For example, one reason for NSSI behavior may be to regulate emotion and elicit attention (Jacobson & Gould, 2007). Students may deliberately harm themselves to feel better (i.e., to "protect" themselves from an even more distressing pain), to get quick relief from upsetting thoughts and feelings, to reclaim a sense of personal control, and/or as a symptom of a mental disorder. Correlates of NSSI include a history of sexual abuse, depression, anxiety, alexithymia (difficulty in experiencing, expressing, and describing emotional reactions), hostility, smoking, dissociation, suicidal ideation, and suicidal behaviors (Jacobson & Gould).

Assisting Students At-Risk for and Engaging in SIB

School counselors need to remain up-to-date with the emerging SIB literature, as there are currently few proven prevention or intervention methods for reducing suicidal and nonsuicidal SIBs (Lieberman, Toste, & Heath, 2009; Prinstein, 2008; Yates, Tracy, & Luthar, 2008). There is some clinical evidence that cognitive-behavioral and problem-solving treatment approaches are effective in reducing SIB (Craigen & Foster, 2009). Although school counselors report feeling underprepared to deal with self-injury (Roberts-Dobie & Donatelle, 2007), supporting students at risk for SIB is based more on professional intuition and "clinical" experience than on well-documented school counseling activities and services. Obviously, deliberate self-injury, like many serious mental health concerns, is a dangerous condition and beyond the scope of school counseling practice and must to be referred out to a highly trained therapist. This section, however, provides some basic school counseling-related activities to assist students and their families.

Prevention   School-based methods to prevent and support students who are at-risk for SIB are not well documented. However, here are a few key recommendations that may work.

1. *Start early.* Beginning with early elementary school children and later reinforced in secondary students, counselor educational activities should address the development of emotion regulation (ER) skills; by doing so, they may well serve to prevent later emotional disorders such as SIB (Ross et al., 2009).

2. *Teach fundamental emotion regulation skills.* Because ER is closely linked with emerging healthy psychosocial functioning as well as early academic success

(Graziano, Reavis, Keane, & Calkins, 2007), students need to learn effective strategies to identify and manage their levels of stress and emotionality. In particular, classroom guidance and small groups should address with students how to manage and cope more productively with increasing levels of arousal, anxiety, and confusing emotions.

3. *Strengthen educator-student relationships.* Elementary and secondary school counselors need to work closely with educators to enhance the student-teacher relationships. Evidence suggests that students with better ER skills have more positive and caring relationships with educators and exhibit fewer behavioral problems (Graziano et al. 2007). In other words, the quality of the student-teacher relationship seems to mediate the relation between children's ER skills and academic achievement.

4. *Screen.* As with depression and anxiety, screening for SIB may be developed in consultation with outside mental health experts. Something paralleling the Systematic Screening for Behavior Disorders process discussed earlier may be helpful model to implement.

Plan Supportive Interventions   Perhaps the most important steps for addressing students who are suspected of or who are already self-harming are listed here.

1. *Notification.* Assuming the SIB was discovered at school, with the ethical and legal considerations (see White Kress, Drouhard, & Costin, 2006, for an excellent review) in mind, the school counselor notifies all relevant parties (e.g., administrator, school nurse, parent/guardian).

2. *Consultation and referral.* Then, in consultation with all appropriate persons, a referral is made within one day (hopefully sooner) to a mental professional who has extensive experience with students with SIB. Depending upon the severity of the wounds, a physician may also be contacted. Diagnosis and prognosis are left to qualified clinicians. In the best-case scenario, determination of whether the student is presenting signs of nonsuicidal (NSSI) or suicidal self-jury (SSI) is shared with the school "point person" (e.g., school counselor), so that appropriate care and follow-up can occur. Ensure that the outside professional(s) has written consent from the parents or guardians to regularly connect with the school counselor.

3. *Collaboration.* Team up with the mental health professional(s), family, and school nurse as well as relevant educators to provide an accommodating and safe school environment. Because teachers have considerable influence on students who self-harm, the teacher-student interaction patterns should be "monitored." Counselors as *liaisons* may need to assist teachers with setting and maintaining realistic classroom academic and behavioral expectations (Malikow, 2006; Roberts-Dobie & Donatelle, 2007). Related to the liaison role, the school counselor can also act as a *coordinator* of support services, working to create school environments where self-injury is more likely to be identified early on by school staff, students, and parents, and students in an early phase of SIB will more readily receive outside counseling

(Roberts-Dobie & Donatelle). The school counselor coordinates the development and implementation of an "action plan" so that all parties are collaborating in the most helpful manner, especially when a student returns to the school from any in-patient treatment facility. As with supporting students with depression and/or anxiety issues, a PBS system can be implemented as well (Doll & Cummings, 2008; Galassi & Akos, 2007; Merchant et al., 2009). Until the student is in a solid recovery stage, school personnel should try to minimize stressful experiences.

4. *Follow-up meetings.* Periodic "check-ins" with the student and family are recommended. With family and student authorization, continue to provide support to other educators (e.g., teachers, coaches) on how to best assist the student. Follow up on the plan and modify it as needed. Assuming the student continues with outpatient therapy while attending classes, consult with the outside professional to determine if additional scaffolding services are needed.

5. *Individual supportive counseling.* Borrowing from Craigen and Foster (2009), when meeting with students one-to-one, several counseling skills have been reported to be most supportive: respectful attending, empathetic understanding, and acting as a friend (i.e., establishing a positive personal connection with the student). Counterproductive counselor behaviors are obviously showing a lack of care and forcing views on clients.

SUMMARY

This chapter has surveyed the major characteristics of anxiety, depression, and self-injurious behavior, three mental health challenges experienced by school-age children and youth. Various research-based approaches were also discussed which professional school counselors can use to assist students with internalizing behavior disorders. School counselors are encouraged to adopt a school-wide or systems-ecological approach to prevention and intervention (Abrams et al., 2005; Doll & Cummings, 2008; Mazza & Reynolds, 2008), which also includes a strengths-based orientation (Galassi & Akos, 2007) and perhaps even a "response to intervention" (RTI; Martinez & Nellis, 2008) framework. An effective comprehensive school counseling program should include the implementation of a positive support system, where students who require extra assistance will receive it within a caring learning community (Sink & Edwards, 2008). An extensive screening plan and school-wide and classroom prevention activities should be instituted as well. When students are identified with emerging anxiety, depression, and/or SIB, specific interventions might be instituted as needed, including immediate referral to an outside child-adolescent psychotherapy/psychiatrist, peer helping and support groups, small group and individual counseling, and supportive collaboration with family members and relevant school personnel. By following this chapter's "best practice" recommendations and reviewing the additional resources provided in Table 3.3, the school counselor can help these troubled children and youth, in time, experience the positive emotional-social and educational outcomes they deserve.

T A B L E   3.3   **Additional Resources for Childhood and Adolescent Depression, Anxiety, and SIB**

Depression and Anxiety

- Abela, J. R., & Hankin, B. J. (Eds.). (2008). *Handbook of depression in children and adolescents.* New York: Guilford.

- Antony, M. M., & Stein, M. B. (Eds). (2009). *Oxford handbook of anxiety and related disorders.* New York: Oxford University Press.

- Evans, D. L., & Andrews, L. W. (2005). *If your adolescent has depression or bipolar disorder: An essential resource for parents.* New York: Oxford University Press. (See Chapter 3: Getting the best treatment for your teen: Medications, Therapy, and More)

- Foa, E. B., & Andrews, L. W. (2006). *If your adolescent has an anxiety disorder: An essential resource for parents.* New York: Oxford University Press.

- Glicken, M. D. (2009). *Evidence-based practice with emotionally troubled children and adolescents.* San Diego, CA: Academic Press.

- Mental Health Association of America. http://www.nmha.org/ (covers emotional disorders in useful and readable language).

- Merrill, K. (2008). *Helping students overcome depression and anxiety: A practical guide.* New York: Guilford.

- National Institute of Mental Health (NIMH). (2009). *Mental health topics.* Retrieved May 21, 2009, from http://www.nimh.nih.gov/health/topics/ (provides valuable general information).

- Rey, J. M., & Birmaher, B. (Eds.). (2009). *Treating child and adolescent depression.* Baltimore, MD: Lippincott Williams & Wilkins.

- Williams, K., & Lebrun, M. (2009). *Keeping kids safe, healthy, and smart.* Landham, MD: Rowman and Littlefield Education.

Self-injurious Behavior[4]

- Walsh, B. W. (2008). *Treating self-injury: A practical guide.* New York: Guildford.

Informational and Factual Web Sites

- American Academy of Child & Adolescent Psychiatry, www.aacap.org/page.ww?name=Self-injury+In+Adolescents&section=Facts+for+Families

- American Association for Marriage and Family Therapy, www.aamft.org/families/Consumer_Updates/Adolescent_Self_Harm.asp

- American Self-Harm Clearinghouse, www.selfinjury.org/

- Helpguide.org, www.helpguide.org/mental/self_injury.htm

- HealthyPlace.com, www.concernedcounseling.com/communities/Self_Injury/Site/index.htm

- Lysamena Project (religious-based information), www.self-injury.org/

- Mayo Clinic, www.mayoclinic.com/health/self-injury/DS00775

(Continued)

---

[4]Web sites were reviewed and recommended by Moyer, Haberstroh, and Marbach (2008); see other highly regarded web sites listed in the reference section.

T A B L E 3.3   **Additional Resources for Childhood and Adolescent Depression, Anxiety, and SIB (Continued)**

- National Center for PTSD, www.ncptsd.va.gov/facts/problems/fs_self_harm.html
- The Prevention Researcher, www.tpronline.org/articles.cfm?articleID=97
- By Parents for Parents, www.byparents-forparents.com/cutting.html
- Right Health.com, www.righthealth.com/search?t=vhealth.all&out=health-goog-sb&lid=goog-ads-sb&q=teen%20cutting%20themselves&o=classic&v=Health
- S.A.F.E. Alternatives, http://www.safe-alternatives.com/
- Self-Injury and Related Issues, www.siari.co.uk/

Supportive Self-Help Web Sites
- Secret Shame, www.palace.net/~llama/psych/injury.html
- LifeSigns, www.selfharm.org/what/index.html
- Crescent Life, Self Injury: www.crescentlife.com/psychissues/self-injury.htm
- Self-Injury Information and Support, www.psyke.org/
- Men Who Self-Injure, formen 10.tripod.com/index.html
- Can't Scream, Can't Shout, www.angelfire.com/grrl/glassangel/
- Self-Injury: A Struggle, http://self-injury.net/
- Self Injury, www.mirror-mirror.org/selfinj.htm

REFERENCES

Abrams, L., Flood, J., & Phelps, L. (2006). Psychopharmacology in the schools. *Psychology in the Schools, 43,* 493–501.

Abrams, K., Theberge, S. K., & Karan, O. C. (2005). Children and adolescents who are depressed: An ecological approach. *Professional School Counseling, 8,* 284–292.

American Academy of Child & Adolescent Psychiatry. (2008). *The depressed child.* Retrieved May 17, 2009, from http://aacap.org/page.ww?section=Facts+for+Families&name=The+Depressed+Child.

American Psychiatric Association. (2000). *Diagnostic and statistical manual of mental disorders* (Text Rev., 4th ed.). Washington, D.C.: Author.

American School Counselor Association. (2005). *ASCA's national model: A foundation for school counseling programs.* Alexandria, VA: Author.

Anderson, E. R., & Hope, D. A. (2008). A review of the tripartite model for understanding the link between anxiety and depression in youth. *Clinical Psychology Review, 28,* 275–287.

Auger, R. (2005). School-based interventions for students with depressive disorders. *Professional School Counseling, 8,* 344–352.

Avenevoli, S. Knight, E., Kessler, R. C., & Merikangas, K. R. (2008). Epidemiology of depression in children and adolescents. In J. R. Z. Abela & B. L. Hankin (Eds.), *Handbook of depression in children and adolescents* (pp. 6–32). New York: Guildford.

Bambara, L. M., & Kern, L. (Eds.). (2005). *Individualized supports for students with problem behaviors: Designing positive behavior plans.* New York: Guilford.

Baginsky, M. (2004). Peer support: Expectations and realities. *Pastoral Care in Education, 22,* 3–9.

Barrett, P. M., & Pahl, K. M. (2006). School-based intervention: Examining a universal approach to anxiety management. *Australian Journal of Guidance & Counselling, 16,* 55–75.

Burns, K. M., & Hulusi, H. M. (2005). Bridging the gap a learning support centre and school: A solution-focused group approach. *Educational Psychology in Practice, 21,* 123–130.

Carr, E. G. (2007). The expanding vision of positive behavior support: Research perspectives on happiness, helpfulness, hopefulness. *Journal of Positive Behavior Interventions, 9,* 3–14.

Colman, I., Wadsworth, M. E. J., Croudace, T. J., & Jones, P. B. (2007). Forty-year psychiatric outcomes following assessment for internalizing disorder in adolescence. *American Journal of Psychiatry, 164,* 126–133.

Craigen, L. M., & Foster, V. (2009). "It was like a partnership of the two of us against the cutting": Investigating the counseling experiences of young adult women who self-injure. *Journal of Mental Health Counseling, 31,* 76–94.

Centers for Disease Control and Prevention. (2005). Mental health in the United States: Health care and well being of children with chronic emotional, behavioral, or developmental problems. *MMWR Weekly, 54,* 985–989.

Cuijpers, P., Straten, A., Smits, N., & Smit, F. (2006). Screening and early psychological intervention for depression in schools: Systematic review and meta-analysis. *European Child & Adolescent Psychiatry, 15,* 300–307.

Curry, J. F., & Reinecke, M. A. (2003). Modular therapy for adolescents with major depression. In M. A. Reinecke, F. M. Dattilio, & A. Freeman (Eds.), *Cognitive therapy with children and adolescents: A casebook for clinical practice* (2nd ed., pp. 95–127). New York: Guildford.

Doll, B., & Cummings, J. A. (Eds.). (2008). *Transforming school mental health services population-based approaches to promoting the competency and wellness of children.* Thousand Oaks, CA: Corwin.

Dollarhide, C. T., & Saginak, K. A. (2008). *Comprehensive school counseling programs: K–12 delivery systems in action.* Boston: Pearson.

Drop, J., & Block, T. (2004). High school peer mentoring that works! *Teaching Exceptional Children, 37,* 56–62.

Dunlap, G., Carr, E. G., Horner, R. H., Zarcone, J. R., & Schwartz, I. (2008). Positive behavior support and applied behavior analysis: A familial alliance. *Behavior Modification, 32,* 682–698.

Dwyer, K. P. (2002). Mental health in the schools. *Journal of Child and Family Studies, 11,* 101–111.

Erford, B. (2007). The Screening Test for Emotional Problems: Studies of reliability and validity. *Measurement and Evaluation in Counseling and Development, 39,* 209–225.

Flannery-Schroeder, E. C. (2006). Reducing anxiety to prevent depression. *American Journal of Preventive Medicine, 31,* S136–S142.

Forum on Child and Family Statistics. (2008). *America's children in brief: Key national indicators of well-being, 2008. Parental reports of emotional and behavioral difficulties.* Retrieved May 10, 2009, from http://childstats.gov/americaschildren

Galassi, J. P., & Akos, P. (2007). *Strengths–based school counseling.* Mahweh, NJ: Lawrence Erlbaum.

Gillham, J. E., Reivich, K. J., Freres, D. R., Chaplin, T. M., Shatte, A. J., Samuels, B., et al. (2007). School-based prevention of depressive symptoms: A randomized controlled study of the effectiveness and specificity of Penn Resiliency Program. *Journal of Consulting and Clinical Psychology, 75,* 9–19.

Gillham, J. E., Shatte, A. J., & Freres, D. R. (2000). Preventing depression: A review of cognitive-behavioral and family interventions. *Applied & Preventive Psychology, 9,* 63–88.

Graziano, R. A., Reavis, R. D., Keane, S. P., & Calkins, S. D. (2007). The role of emotion regulation in children's early academic success. *Journal of School Psychology, 45,* 3–19.

Gysbers, N. C., & Henderson, P. (2006). *Developing and managing your school guidance and counseling program* (4th ed.). Alexandria, VA: American Counseling Association.

Handler, M. W., Rey, J., Connell, J., Thier, K., Feinberg, A., & Putnam, R. (2007). Practical considerations in creating school-wide positive behavior support in public schools. *Psychology in the Schools, 44,* 29–39.

Heath, N. L., Schaub, K., Holly, S., & Nixon, M. K. (2009). Self-injury: Review of population and clinical studies in adolescents. In M. K. Nixon & N. L. Heath (Eds.), *Self-injury in youth: The essential guide to assessment and intervention* (pp. 9–28). New York: Routledge.

Horowitz, J. L., & Garber, J. (2006). The prevention of depressive symptoms in children and adolescents: A meta-analytic review. *Journal of Consulting and Clinical Psychology, 74,* 401–415.

InCrisis. (2007). *Online behavioral evaluations & reports: The prevalence of mental health and addictive disorders.* Retrieved April 13, 2009, from http://www.incrisis.org/Articles/PrevalenceMHProblems.htm.

Jacobson, C. M., & Gould, M. (2007). The epidemiology and phenomenology of non-suicidal self-injurious behavior among adolescents: A critical review of the literature. *Archives of Suicide Research, 11,* 129–47.

Kendall, P. C., Hedtke, K. A., & Aschenbrand, S. G. (2006). Anxiety disorders. In D. A. Wolfe & E. J. Mash (Eds.), *Behavioral and emotional disorders in adolescents* (pp. 259–299). New York: Guilford.

Kessler, R. C., Berglund, P. A., Demler, O., Jin, R., & Walters, E. E. (2005). Lifetime prevalence and age-of-onset distributions of DSM–IV disorders in the National Comorbidity Survey Replication (NCS–R). *Archives of General Psychiatry, 62,* 593–602.

Klonsky, E. D. (2007). The functions of deliberate self-injury. A review of the evidence. *Clinical Psychology Review, 27,* 226–239.

Klonsky, E. D., & Glenn, C. R. (2009). Psychosocial risk and protective factors. In M. K. Nixon & N. L. Heath (Eds.), *Self-injury in youth: The essential guide to assessment and intervention* (pp. 45–58). New York: Routledge.

Kramer, U., & Zimmermann, G. (2009). Fear and anxiety at the basis of adolescent externalizing and internalizing behaviors. *International Journal of Offender Therapy and Comparative Criminology, 53,* 113–120.

Kress, V. E., Gibson, D. M., & Reynolds, C. A. (2004). Adolescents who self-injure: Implications and strategies for school counselors. *Professional School Counseling, 7,* 195–201.

Laye-Gindhu, A., & Schonert-Reichl, K. A. (2005). Nonsuicidal self-harm among community adolescents: Understanding the "whats" and "whys" of self-harm. *Journal of Youth and Adolescence, 34,* 447–457.

Levitt, J. L., Sansone, R. A., & Cohn, L. (Eds.). (2004). *Self-harm and eating disorders: Dynamics, assessment, and treatment.* New York: Brunner-Routledge.

Lewis, M. W., & Lewis, A. C. (1996). Peer helping programs: Helper role, supervisor training, and suicidal behavior. *Journal of Counseling & Development, 74,* 307–13.

Lieberman, R. A., Toste, J. R., & Heath, N. L. (2009). Nonsuicidal self-injury in the schools: Prevention and intervention. In M. K. Nixon & N. L. Heath (Eds.), *Self-injury in youth: The essential guide to assessment and intervention* (pp. 195–216). New York: Routledge.

Lloyd-Richardson, E. E., Nock, M. K., & Prinstein, M. L. (2009). Functions of adolescent nonsuicidal self-injury. In M. K. Nixon & N. L. Heath (Eds.), *Self-injury in youth: The essential guide to assessment and intervention* (pp. 29–41). New York: Routledge.

Malikow, M. (2006). When students cut themselves. *Education Digest, 71,* 45–50.

Martinez, R. S., & Nellis, L. M. (2008). Response to intervention. A school-wide approach for the promotion of academic wellness in students. In B. Doll & J. A.Cummings (Eds.), *Transforming school mental health services population-based approaches to promoting the competency and wellness of children* (pp. 143–164). Thousand Oaks, CA: Corwin.

Masia-Warner, C., Nangle, D. W., & Hansen, D. J. (2006). Bringing evidence-based child mental health services to the schools: General issues and specific populations. *Education and Treatment of Children, 29,* 165–172.

Mazza, J. J., & Reynolds, W. M. (2008). School-wide approaches to the prevention and intervention for depression and suicidal behaviors. In B. Doll & J. A.Cummings (Eds.), *Transforming school mental health services population-based approaches to promoting the competency and wellness of children* (pp. 213–241). Thousand Oaks, CA: Corwin.

McWhirter, B. T., & Burrow, J. J. (2001). Assessment and treatment recommendations for children and adolescents with depression. In E. R. Welfel & R. E. Ingersoll (Eds.), *The mental health desk reference: A practice-based guide to diagnosis, treatment, and professional ethics* (pp. 199–204). Hoboken, NJ: John Wiley.

Merchant, M., Anderson, D. H., Caldarella, P., Fisher, A., Young, B. J., & Young, K. R. (2009). Schoolwide screening and programs of positive behavior support: Informing universal interventions. *Preventing School Failure, 53,* 131–144.

Merrill, K. M. (2008). *Behavioral, social, and emotional assessment of children and adolescents* (3rd ed.). New York: Lawrence Erlbaum.

Morgan, P. L., Farkas, G., & Wu, Q. (2009). Kindergarten predictors of recurring externalizing and internalizing psychopathology in the third and fifth grades. *Journal of Emotional and Behavioral Disorders, 17*(2), 67–79.

Moyer, M., Haberstroh, S., & Marbach, C. (2008). Self-injurious behaviors on the net: A survey of resources for school counselors. *Professional School Counseling, 11,* 277–284.

Murray, L., Creswell, C., & Cooper, P. J. (2009). The development of anxiety disorders in childhood: An integrative review. *Psychological Medicine.* Retrieved May 24, 2009, from http://journals.cambridge.org/action/displayAbstract?aid=4031752#.

National Alliance on Mental Illness. (2009). *Early-onset depression.* Retrieved May 20, 2009, from http://www.nami.org/Content/ContentGroups/Helpline1/Facts_About_Childhood_Depression.htm.

National Dissemination Center for Children with Disabilities (NICHCY). (2004, January). *Disability fact sheet (No. 5): Emotional disturbance.* Washington, D.C.: Author. Retrieved April 30, 2009, from http://www.nichcy.org/InformationResources/Documents/NICHCY%20PUBS/fs5.pdf.

National Institute of Mental Health. (2009). *What is a depressive disorder?* Retrieved May 16, 2009, from http://www.nimh.nih.gov/publicat/depression.cfm#ptdep1.

Nixon, M. K., & Heath, N. L. (Eds.). (2009). *Self-injury in youth: The essential guide to assessment and intervention.* New York: Routledge.

Nock, M. K., Joiner, T. E., Gordon, K. H., Lloyd-Richardson, E., & Prinstein, M. J. (2006). Non-suicidal self-injury among adolescents: Diagnostic correlates and relation to suicide attempts. *Psychiatry Research, 144,* 65–72.

Nock, M. K., & Prinstein, M. J. (2005). Contextual features and behavioral function of self-mutilation and among adolescents. *Journal of Abnormal Psychology, 114,* 140–146.

Osuch, E. A., & Payne, G. W. (2009). Neurobiological perspectives on self-injury. In M. K. Nixon & N. L. Heath (Eds.), *Self-injury in youth: The essential guide to assessment and intervention* (pp. 79–110). New York: Routledge.

Oswald, D. P., & Mazefskey, C. A. (2006). Empirically supported psychotherapy interventions for internalizing disorders. *Psychology in the Schools, 43,* 439–449.

Poulou, M. (2005). The prevention of emotional and behavioural difficulties in schools: Teachers' suggestions. *Educational Psychology in Practice, 21,* 37–52.

Prinstein, M. J. (2008). Introduction to the special section on suicide and nonsuicidal self-injury: A review of unique challenges and important directions for self-injury science. *Journal of Consulting and Clinical Psychology, 76,* 1–8.

Reddy, L. A., Newman, E., De Courtney, A. T., & Chun, V. (2009). Effectiveness of school-based prevention and intervention programs for children and adolescents with emotional disturbance: A meta-analysis. *Journal of School Psychology, 47,* 77–99.

Reddy, L. A., & Richardson, L. (2006). School-based prevention and intervention programs for children with emotional disturbance. *Education and Treatment of Children, 29,* 379–404.

Roberts-Dobie, S., & Donatelle, R. J. (2007). School counselors and student self-injury. *Journal of School Health, 77,* 257–264.

Rodham, K., & Hawton, K. (2009). Epidemiology and phenomenology of nonsuicidal self-injury. In M. K. Nock (Eds.), *Understanding nonsuicidal self-injury: Origins, assessment, and treatment* (pp. 37–62). Washington, D.C.: American Psychological Association.

Ross, S., Heath, N. L., & Toste, J. R. (2009). *American Journal of Orthopsychiatry, 79,* 83–92.

Roza, S. J., Hofstra, M. B., van der Ende, J., & Verhulst, F. C. (2003). Stable prediction of mood and anxiety disorders based on behavioral and emotional problems in childhood: A 14-year follow-up during childhood, adolescence, and young adulthood. *American Journal of Psychiatry, 160,* 2116–2121.

Rudolph, K. D., Hammen, C., & Daley, S. E. (2006). Mood disorders. In D. A. Wolfe & E. J. Mash (Eds.), *Behavioral and emotional disorders in adolescents* (pp. 300–342). New York: Guilford.

Safrin, S. P. (2006). Using the effective behavior supports survey to guide development of schoolwide positive behavior support. *Journal of Positive Behavior Interventions, 8,* 3–9.

Sansone, R. A., & Levitt, J. L. (2005). Borderline personality and eating disorders. *Eating Disorders: The Journal of Treatment & Prevention, 13,* 71–83.

Sink, C. A., & Igelman, C. N. (2004). Anxiety disorders. In F. M. Kline & L. B. Silver (Eds.), *The educator's guide to mental health issues in the classroom* (pp. 171–191). Baltimore, MD: Paul H. Brookes.

Sink, C. A., & Edwards, C. (2008). Supportive learning communities and the transformative role of professional school counselors. *Professional School Counseling, 12,* 108–114.

Slater, P., & McKeown, M. (2004). The role of peer counseling and support in helping to reduce anxieties around transition from primary to secondary school. *Counselling and Psychotherapy Research, 4,* 72–79.

Sommers-Flanagan, R., Barrett-Hakanson, T., Clarke, C., & Sommers-Flanagan, J. (2000). A psychoeducational school-based coping and social skills group for depressed students. *Journal for Specialists in Group Work, 25,* 170–190.

Substance Abuse and Mental Health Services Administration's (SAMHSA) National Mental Health Information Center. (2003). *Major depression in children and adolescents.* Retrieved May 21, 2009, from http://mentalhealth.samhsa.gov/publications/allpubs/Ca-0011/default.asp.

Tobias, A. K. (2001). Prevention: A practical approach to preventing violence in elementary schools. In D. S. Sandhu (Ed.), *Elementary school counseling in the new millennium* (pp. 159–169). Alexandria, VA: American Counseling Association.

U.S. Department of Education. (2004). *Public Law 108–446 Individuals With Disabilities Act.* Retrieved May 21, 2009, from http://frwebgate.access.gpo.gov/cgi-bin/getdoc.cgi?dbname=108_cong_public_laws&docid=f:publ446.108.

U.S. Department of Education. (2009). *Protecting students with disabilities: Frequently asked questions about section 504 and the education of children with disabilities.* Retrieved May 21, 2009, from http://www.ed.gov/about/offices/list/ocr/504faq.html safeguards.

U.S. Department of Health and Human Services. (1999). *Mental health: A report of the Surgeon General.* Rockville, MD: U.S. Department of Health and Human Services, Substance Abuse and Mental Health Services Administration, Center for Mental Health Services, National Institutes of Health, National Institute of Mental Health. Retrieved May 21, 2009, from http://www.surgeongeneral.gov/library/mentalhealth/home.html.

U.S. Public Health Service. (2000). *Report of the Surgeon General's Conference on Children's Mental Health: A national action agenda.* Washington, D.C.: Department of Health and Human Services. Retrieved May 21, 2009, from http://www.surgeongeneral.gov/topics/cmh/childreport.html.

Walker, H. M., Severson, H. H., Nicholson, F., Kehle, T., Jenson, W. R., & Clark, E. (1994). Replication of the Systematic Screening for Behavior Disorders (SSBD) procedure for the identification of at-risk children. *Journal of Emotional and Behavioral Disorders, 2,* 66–77.

Walsh, F. (2006). *Strengthening family resilience* (2nd ed.). New York: Guilford.

Weist, M. D., Rubin, M., Moore, E., Adelsheim, S., & Wrobel, G. (2007). Mental health screening in schools. *Journal of School Health, 77,* 53–58.

Weisz, J. R., McCarty, C. A., & Valeri, S. M. (2006). Effects of psychotherapy for Depression in children and adolescents: A meta-analysis. *Psychological Bulletin, 132,* 132–149.

White Kress, V. E., Drouhard, N., & Costin, A. (2006). Students who self-injure school counselor ethical and legal considerations. *Professional School Counseling, 10,* 203–209.

Wolfe, D. A., & Mash, E. J. (Eds.). (2006). *Behavioral and emotional disorders in adolescents: Nature, assessment, and treatment.* New York: Guilford.

Yates, T. M., Tracy, A. J., & Luthar, S. S. (2008). Nonsuicidal self-injury among "privileged" youths: Longitudinal and cross-sectional approaches to developmental process. *Journal of Consulting and Clinical Psychology, 76,* 52–62.

YouthNet. (2009). *Self-harm: Recovery, advice, and support.* Retrieved May 25, 2009, from http://www.thesite.org/healthandwellbeing/mentalhealth/selfharm.

Chapter 4

Eating Disorders, Obesity, and Body Image Concerns

Prevention and Intervention

ANGELA D. BARDICK, SHELLY
RUSSELL-MAYHEW, KERRY B. BERNES
AND JENNIFER I. BERNES

**Registered Psychologist, University of Calgary,
University of Lethbridge, and Registered Psychologist**

I t is important for professional school counselors to be concerned about students' health and wellness. They may even encounter elementary-age children who seem excessively worried about their weight and body shape (Cavanaugh & Lemberg, 1999; Haines, Neumark-Sztainer, & Thiel, 2007). The challenges of childhood and adolescent obesity and eating disorders (Butryn & Wadden, 2005; Russell-Mayhew, 2006) are discussion topics of health news around the world (e.g., Jensen, 2009; Monro & Gail, 2005) and drastic actions by educational policymakers (National Association of State Boards of Education & Pekruhn, 2009). School counselors are in an ideal position to implement school-based prevention programs, identify at-risk individuals, make appropriate referrals for intervention or treatment, and support students who may be recovering from eating disorders (Akos & Levitt, 2002; Choate, 2007). This chapter provides an overview of eating disorders within a school environment, a case study, a problem description, and practical evidence-based interventions that may be implemented in the school setting.

If school counselors listened to student and teacher discussions in classrooms, hallways, and teachers' lounges, they might be surprised at how much time is spent talking about bodies—their weight, size, and shape, what food to put into or not put into them, how to move them, and how people believe they "should" look (i.e., thin and muscular) or "should not" look (i.e., fat). Counselors would likely hear compliments about weight loss and teasing about weight gain (Kostanski & Gullone, 2007). They may see "skinny" children, "fat" children, and "ugly" children being bullied. School counselors would also typically see students being admired for their athletic prowess (e.g., "athlete of the year" awards) and physical beauty, and other children being shunned for not being athletically adept (e.g., students who are picked last for teams). There is often much talk in the cafeteria and lunch rooms about food—what to eat and not to eat, diet advice, and how "I wish I could eat like so-and-so and not gain weight." Students may talk about celebrities' bodies and compare their bodies to current standards of physical beauty. School counselors may occasionally hear wishful thinking ("I wish I was as tall/lean/thin/muscular/strong/beautiful, etc. as him/her"). They also may be drawn into conversations with students who are talking about themselves negatively.

If school counselors observed student and teacher behaviors (e.g., McVey, Gusella, Tweed, & Ferrari, 2009), they may see subtle and overt ways in which students are taught about their bodies and culturally "acceptable" weight and shape. For example, students are often weighed and measured in physical education and health classes for the purpose of teaching about physical health and well-being. Healthy body weight and healthy eating are often taught as topics in health, science, and food studies or nutrition classes. Regrettably, talk about weight and illnesses related to weight (i.e., eating disorders) that is considered "educational" may adversely affect students' perceptions of their bodies and of themselves (Russell & Ryder, 2001a; Steiner-Adair, 1994). The risks of focusing on illness and disorder in the school setting are that students may learn risky behaviors from the descriptions of problems and develop unhealthy attitudes and behaviors that lead to or exacerbate body image dissatisfaction and disordered eating and exercise behaviors (Russell & Ryder; Steiner-Adair).

What school counselors cannot observe are students' negative thoughts about weight, body shape, size, and food, or their private behaviors. For example, counselors will not usually be aware of which students throw out their lunches and drink diet soda because they believe they need to lose weight; wear baggy clothes because believe they have to hide their bodies; use steroids

Mia: A School-Based Case Study

Mia is a 15-year-old female starting Grade 10 at a new high school. She received good grades during elementary and junior high school, and teachers often compliment her for being a "model student." She comes from a stable and secure family background. She is involved in piano lessons, and is an accomplished singer. She has a part-time job at the local library, and is physically active by biking, rollerblading, and taking her dog for walks. But Mia has a secret. She hates her body, and desperately wants to be thinner. She wakes half an hour early each morning to do 100 each of sit-ups, push-ups, and leg lifts. She no longer enjoys walking her dog, but does it twice a day to "burn off more calories." She has decided to become a vegetarian, not because of her beliefs about eating meat, but to cut out "extra" calories and fat. She has also vowed to throw out half her lunch each day and drink a diet soda instead. She spends class time planning and evaluating her diet and exercise programs, and avoids social activities because she does not want to eat in front of others. She weighs herself before breakfast, after breakfast, after school, and before bed. She cries herself to sleep because the number on the scale is not decreasing. She compares her body size to other girls at school and believes she does not have friends because she is fat. Mia's family and friends think it is "just a phase" and often compliment her on her "healthy choices." Mia may not meet the criteria for a diagnosable eating disorder, but her over-concern with weight, diet, exercise, and hatred of her body is a significant concern.

to enhance their muscle mass and athletic ability; join athletic clubs as a means to lose weight; spend hours calculating their caloric and fat intake instead of doing homework or having fun with friends and family; obsess about their weight and body to the point of developing an eating disorder; or have "given up" and are apathetic about their physical health and well-being. Take the case study of Mia, above, for example.

OVERVIEW AND CHARACTERISTICS OF
EATING DISORDERS

Within the school environment, students' individual perceptions of their bodies and others' bodies vary greatly, ranging from one extreme of complacency to another extreme of obsession with one's body. Some students may ignore the importance of caring for their bodies and develop unhealthy habits (e.g., smoking, drinking alcohol, drug use, poor nutrition) while other students may take their physical appearance far too seriously and develop unhealthy habits in an attempt to change the appearance of their bodies (e.g., food restriction, over-exercise). Some students may learn to dislike exercise because they do not excel in sports, while other students may take their participation in sports too seriously and harm themselves while striving to "be the best" (e.g., overtraining and steroid use). Some students may develop eating disorders (e.g., anorexia, bulimia, binge eating disorder) or related body image disorders (e.g., muscle dysmorphia), while other students may feel badly about their bodies and show an over-concern with their weight and body shape but not demonstrate full-blown eating disorder symptoms. Unless attended to in some way by the school, students may continue a pattern of attitudes and behaviors towards their bodies and others' bodies that contribute to body dislike, unhealthy body-related behaviors, and an attitude that it is acceptable to comment on, tease, and judge their own body and other people's bodies.

Subtypes, Prevalence, and Long-Term Outcomes

With the typical onset in late adolescence affecting mostly white females (90%; Merrill, 2008), disordered eating is further along the continuum of unhealthy behaviors, and may occur when a number of unhealthy eating and exercise behaviors coincide (e.g., the use of laxatives for weight loss or steroids for increased muscle mass, bingeing, purging, or fasting). Regrettably, because the eating disorders have many overlapping characteristics, school counselors will find the research literature somewhat confusing on how to identify subtypes (Merrill; Thomas, Vartanian, & Brownell, 2009). Dysfunctional eating may lead to eating disorders, such as Binge Eating Disorder (BED; eating enormous amounts of food in short periods of time with no compensatory behaviors), Bulimia Nervosa (BN; binge eating with compensating behaviors such as vomiting, over-exercise, or laxative use), and Anorexia Nervosa (AN; restrictive eating with or without compensatory behaviors). Eating disorders which seem to fall under the general area of internalizing disorders (see Chapter 3) are characterized by multiple symptoms including severe disturbances in eating behaviors and attitudes (Cavanaugh & Lemberg, 1999), weight and body shape preoccupation, impulsivity (Boisseau, Thompson-Brenner, Eddy, & Satir, 2009), and fear of fat (American Psychiatric Association [APA], 2000b; Levitt, 2003). Muscle dysmorphia may also be considered a serious body image disorder, in which individuals engage in excessive exercise and other compensating behaviors (i.e., steroid use) in an attempt to build muscle (Pope, Phillips, & Olivardia, 2000). For a more detailed summary of clinical dimensions of eating disorders, readers might peruse Yager and Powers's (2007) and Smolak and Thompson's (2008) comprehensive texts.

Eating disorders may become chronic, life-threatening conditions with devastating physical, emotional, and behavioral consequences (Lask & Bryant-Waugh, 1999; Steinhausen, 2009). For example, for AN, Steinhausen's summary of outcome studies suggest that there is an 18-fold increase in mortality among sufferers, including a high suicide rate, approximately 20% of sufferers show chronic symptoms, and over 50% of sufferers experience either a complete or a partial eating disorder in combination with another psychiatric disorder, or another psychiatric disorder without an eating disorder. For BN, the overall long-term outcomes are only minimally better. However, the rate of mortality is much lower in this group and the social adjustment and the quality of interpersonal relationships tend to normalize in most cases.

The Academy of Eating Disorders (n.d.) reported that the incidence of eating disorders has increased over the last 30–40 years, with about 0.5% to 1.0% of late adolescent or adult women meeting criteria for AN (see APA's 2000a *Diagnostic and Statistical Manual of Mental Disorders, Fourth Edition, Text Revision;* DSM–IV–TR). Approximately 1.0% to 2.0% of late adolescent and adult women met the criteria for a BN diagnosis. These prevalence rates differ slightly from those reported in the DSM–IV–TR (APA, 2000a), where both AN and BN were found in approximately 0.5% and 0.1% to 0.3% of female samples, respectively, and less than a tenth of that figure among males (APA, 2000a). Both sources thus suggest that diagnosable eating disorders are relatively uncommon. However, the BRIDGE graph discussed in the next section clearly explains that the attitudes and behaviors leading up to them are common (i.e., body dissatisfaction combined with behavioral efforts to change one's body, especially dieting). As noted in our case study, Mia does not currently meet the criteria for a diagnosable eating disorder; however, she clearly demonstrates unhealthy attitudes and behaviors that, if not addressed now, may lead to more serious problems.

The BRIDGE Model of Healthy Versus Unhealthy Body Image

The development of weight and body image concerns may best be described using a continuum of body image attitudes and behaviors that may lead towards health or ill health. Although there are other useful counselor-focused models to draw from (e.g., Choate, 2005), "BRIDGE": *B*uilding the *R*elationship between *B*ody *I*mage and *D*isordered *E*ating *G*raph and *E*xplanation (Russell & Ryder, 2001a; Russell-Mayhew, 2007) is a framework for describing the connection between attitudes individuals may have towards their bodies and the behaviors that they may practice as a result of these attitudes. A brief summary of BRIDGE is provided in Figure 4.1; however, a full explanation of BRIDGE can be found elsewhere (Russell & Ryder, 2001a, 2001b).

BRIDGE is an appropriate framework for understanding the development of body image and eating disorders in school-age children because it encompasses a continuum of body image attitudes and behaviors, ranging from healthy to unhealthy (Russell-Mayhew, 2007). The horizontal axis of the BRIDGE graph describes body image as a continuum that ranges from healthy to unhealthy. Body image may be defined as the mental image a person has of their physical appearance and the attitudes and feelings they have about it (Lutter & Jaffee, 1996). The vertical axis of the BRIDGE graph describes body-related behaviors that range from healthy to unhealthy. The healthiest body image and the healthiest behaviors are nearest the intersect point on the graph and become increasingly unhealthy as the graph moves outward.

According to the BRIDGE model, a healthy body image corresponds with healthy behaviors such as healthy eating (i.e., eating a wide variety of foods according to current guides to healthy eating) and healthy activity (i.e., an active lifestyle). As the graph moves outward, unhealthy body image and behaviors are addressed. For example, when food is used to cope with feelings and not

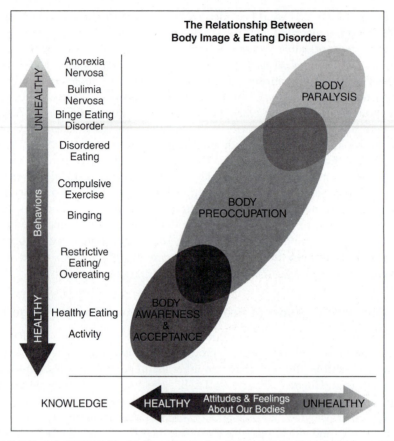

FIGURE 4.1   BRIDGE Model (Russell & Ryder, 2001a, 2001b; Russell-Mayhew, 2007)

consumed in a healthy manner it may lead to restrictive eating (i.e., dieting to control body size), overeating (i.e., natural cues of hunger and fullness are ignored), or bingeing (eating a large quantity of food in a short period of time). Physical activity may also move from healthy to unhealthy when the primary motivation is to control one's body size. For example, a preoccupation with the belief that one's body is not sufficiently lean and muscular may lead to compensating behaviors (i.e., excessive weight lifting and steroid use) that are considered unhealthy. If a school counselor were to use the BRIDGE graph to identify Mia's attitudes and behaviors toward food and exercise, her movement towards an unhealthy body image would be apparent.

The BRIDGE graph further defines the relationship between body image and eating disorders (Russell–Mayhew, 2007). First, *body awareness and acceptance* may accompany healthy attitudes and healthy behaviors when individuals accept their bodies and understand that how they look is only a part of who they are as a whole person. Second, *body preoccupation* may occur when individuals are overly concerned with their body's weight and shape. Body preoccupation may be influenced by the standard of thinness and muscularity that has become a cur-rent beauty ideal along with damaging beliefs about fat (Crandall, 1994; Levitt, 2003). Third, *body paralysis* develops when body preoccupation takes priority over everything else, which may contribute to clinically significant distress or impairment in social and/or occupational functioning (e.g., canceling family engagements in order to work out). The intersection between the most severe unhealthy body image and unhealthy behaviors is most closely connected with eating and body image disorders. According to the BRIDGE graph, Mia in our case study appears to be fluctuating between body preoccupation (excessive con-cern with her weight and shape) and body paralysis (avoiding social activities because of fear of being judged for her size). Should she continue in this manner, it is likely that her unhealthy attitudes and behaviors will interfere with her growth and functioning.

By clearly linking a continuum of body image with a continuum of body-related behaviors, the BRIDGE graph indicates that the prevention of eating disorders requires intervention before attitudes and behaviors start becoming unhealthy. As well, the BRIDGE graph indicates that if increasing unhealthy attitudes and behaviors contribute to eating disorders, then a movement towards body awareness and acceptance may facilitate a return to health.

RECOMMENDATIONS FOR SCHOOL COUNSELING PRACTICE

Eating Disorder Prevention in Schools

School counselors play an important role in the prevention and early identification of eating disorders. They are in a unique position to observe students' attitudes towards food, weight, and body shape; act as positive role models for students; and teach students stress management, problem-solving skills, and the importance of engaging in healthy behaviors (Bardick et al., 2004; Powers & Johnson, 1999; Russell & Ryder, 2001a, 2001b; Smolak, Harris, Levine, & Shisslak, 2001). School counselors need to be active in prevention efforts as well as aware of what to do when an individual student presents with the early warning signs of an eating disorder.

Current eating disorder prevention literature calls for school-based interven-tion programs that focus on the development of healthy attitudes and behaviors that contribute to improved body image and overall well-being in all students (Russell & Ryder, 2001a; Russell-Mayhew, Arthur, & Ewashen, 2007). Neumark-Sztainer et al. (2006) emphasized a need for school programs to limit their focus on information-giving about eating disorders or on detailed descriptions of in-dividuals who have "recovered." Programs that emphasize the signs and symptoms of eating disorders may inadvertently teach dangerous behaviors to impression-able youth (Russell & Ryder, 2001a; Steiner-Adair, 1994). As well, practices such as weighing students and comparing athletic ability among students need to be reconsidered in school programs, as these practices may contribute to the development of unhealthy attitudes and behaviors in regards to body image, food intake, and lifelong exercise. Multidimensional programs that emphasize change at both the individual and school levels have been most effective, and modification of the larger environment is becoming the focus of eating disorder prevention initiatives (Neumark-Sztainer et al., 2006). In this way, the focus is not on a specific at-risk group but rather on promoting healthy messages that benefit all students.

School-Wide Prevention Programs

The primary goals of school-based eating disorder prevention programs should be to challenge current standards of beauty (i.e., thin and muscular), teach critical thinking skills (e.g., examine media messages about the "ideal" body), improve communication and interpersonal skills, encourage tolerance about differences in appearance (i.e., education about weight discrimination), help students develop a healthy body image, and increase self-confidence (Levine, Piran, & Stoddard, 1999; Russell & Ryder, 2001a, 2001b; Russell-Mayhew, 2007). Emphasizing the importance of self-acceptance, positive body image, and healthy eating and exercise behaviors, as noted by the BRIDGE graph (Russell & Ryder, 2001a, 2001b), helps students develop a healthy resistance to eating disorders. Encouraging students to examine and develop strategies for combating the internalization of the "thin ideal" has also been demonstrated as effective (Roehrig, Thompson, Brannick, & van den Berg, 2006). Overall, it is important to teach students how to care for their bodies in healthy ways, to accept their bodies and understand the changes that will occur over time, and understand that the reflection they see in the mirror is not a complete picture of who they are as a whole person. In this regard, eating disorder prevention programs need to begin at early developmental stages (Neumark-Sztainer et al., 2006).

It is crucial for eating disorder prevention programs to teach students the importance of developing acceptance of their own bodies as well as the bodies of others. For example, unhealthy beliefs about obesity may lead to poor peer relationships, discrimination, prejudice, and stigmatization (Klaczynski, Goold, & Mudry, 2004; Russell-Mayhew, 2006). Children whose bodies deviate from the "thin ideal" are likely to be viewed as less physically and socially attractive (Crandall, D'Anello, Sakalli, Wieczorkowski, & Feather, 2001; Thompson & Stice, 2001), which may lead to inappropriate peer rejection, comments, and teasing. In our case study Mia had not been teased about the size or shape of her body, but because she had witnessed the torment other students received about their bodies, she began to believe that she must remain a certain size to avoid social harassment. Discouraging weight and shape teasing/bullying and sexual harassment is critical in promoting acceptance (Smolak, 1999; Steiner-Adair, 1994; Sweetingham & Waller, 2008). The goal is to help both girls and boys in the early grades learn that it is hurtful and unfair to reject their peers because of their skin color, religious background, body size, or physical challenges.

Clearly, early intervention is an important feature of assisting students with eating disorders. With the implementation of the States for Treatment Access and Research (STAR) program by the National Eating Disorders Association (NEDA), which aims to improve the advocacy and early intervention and treatment of eating disorders (Gregorio, 2009), a number of school-based programs focused on developing healthy body-related attitudes and behaviors have been developed, with promising results (Varnado-Sullivan & Horton, 2006). Most prevention programs recognize the multi-faceted nature of eating disorders and body image concerns, and therefore incorporate student, teacher, parent, and community involvement.

- The *Body-Logic Program* (Varnado-Sullivan et al., 2001) is an eating disorder prevention program for adolescents. This program includes an in-class curriculum, teacher workshop, and parent information sessions. The *Body-Logic Program* was shown to have a positive influence on female participants, but not male participants.

- *Planet Health* (Austin, Field, Wiecha, Peterson, & Gortmaker, 2005) is an obesity prevention program targeting disordered eating in adolescent girls. This program uses classroom lessons, teacher training, wellness sessions, and fitness funds to help adolescents focus on increasing physical activity and consumption of fruits and vegetables, and decreasing television viewing and consumption of high fat foods. Program evaluation, which used only female participants in Grades 6 and 7, indicated that female purging behaviors and use of diet pills were reduced.

- *Very Important Kids* (Haines, Neumark-Sztainer, Perry, Hannan, & Levine, 2006) is a multi-component, school-based intervention focused on preventing teasing and unhealthy weight control behaviors. This program is multi-component, with an after-school program, school environment components, and a family component. Program evaluation indicated a reduction in weight-related teasing, but no changes in weight control behaviors.

- *Healthy-Schools, Healthy Kids* (McVey, Tweed, & Blackmore, 2007) is a comprehensive school-based program with a focus on developing media awareness of cultural pressures to obtain a certain body size, understanding natural changes in the body throughout puberty, understanding the negative influence of peer pressure to diet or peer teasing, and stress management and self-esteem building skills. An environmental approach is emphasized, with school staff training, parent education, in-class curriculum, student support group, theatre presentation, focus groups, posters/video presentations, and public service announcements. Program evaluation indicated a positive influence on body satisfaction, reduced internalization of media ideals, decreased disordered eating, but no changes in weight-based teasing or size acceptance.

- Other programs, such as the *Body Image Kits* (Body Image Works, 2005) utilize an environmental approach with student, teacher, parent, and community components and show promise as effective wellness-based prevention programs.

Whichever school-based prevention program is used, the following is a summary of the topics that should be addressed in a school environment:

1. Self-esteem and self-acceptance
2. Critical thinking (e.g., examination of attitudes and beliefs towards obesity and the thin ideal)
3. Self-assertion, communication, and interpersonal skills
4. Tolerance and acceptance of other people's bodies and physical abilities (e.g., inappropriateness of weight-related teasing or comments, the belief that bodies can be healthy at any size)
5. Avoidance of "fat-talk" and "diet-talk" (e.g., comments around weight and food restriction)
6. Influence of the media in perpetuating beliefs in the thin ideal and beliefs about food
7. Strategies for improving body image (e.g., self-care, respect for one's abilities and limitations)
8. Importance of active lifestyles and healthy eating (e.g., eating a variety of foods, paying attention to internal hunger cues, engaging in healthy and enjoyable physical activity)
9. Dangers of trying to change one's body through dieting or other behaviors (e.g., steroid use)
10. Effective skills for dealing with negative emotions and stressors

Overall, a participatory approach is encouraged where all stakeholders (students, parents and teachers) are invested in changes that create a positive environment for every 'body.'

The following topics need not be addressed in a school environment:

1. Specific eating disorders and their causes, without putting them in the context of healthy versus unhealthy attitudes and behaviors
2. Specific behaviors associated with eating disorders (e.g., vomiting, laxative use, etc.), as these may inadvertently encourage individuals to "try out" unhealthy behaviors
3. Teaching students to evaluate their health solely through weight, body measurements, and Body Mass Index, as these can encourage competition and an excess focus on the body.

On the whole, a focus on healthy attitudes and behaviors should dominate over discussion about illness and disorder.

In order to help students move towards healthy body image and behaviors, professional school counselors and other key adults (i.e., teachers, coaches, and parents) who work with children may first need to examine how their own attitudes and behaviors towards weight, dieting, and body image may inadvertently affect the children with which they work (Dohnt & Tiggemann, 2008; Graber, Archibald, & Brooks-Gunn, 1999; Powers & Johnson, 1999; Russell & Ryder, 2001a). For example, Bardick et al. (2004) asserts that "well-intentioned comments about a child's appearance or physical ability and/or ill-considered comments about weight or laziness have the potential to cause serious damage to a child's emerging body image and self concept" (p. 169). It is important for adults who work with children to be role models who reinforce healthy attitudes and behaviors and help students critically examine negative societal messages about body image, perfectionism, and achievement (Vitousek, Watson, & Wilson, 1998). For example, Mia's teachers and parents would be encouraged to examine how their own weight-related attitudes and behaviors may be positively or negatively affecting Mia's body image. Understated forms of body discrimination (or weight-based teasing or bullying) may be undetected or overlooked by parents or teachers if the parents themselves are "fat-phobic" or have bought into contemporary sociocultural ideals of ideal body shape (McVey et al., 2007; Monro & Huon, 2005). Therefore, school-based eating disorder prevention programs should also have an adult psycho-educational component to enhance the school and home environments (Neumark-Sztainer et al., 2006). It does not make sense to encourage students to adapt healthy behaviors and attitudes if the adults who influence their lives continue to diet and make weight-related comments (Russell-Mayhew, Arthur, & Ewashen, in press).

By implementing a school-wide prevention program, where tolerance, acceptance, and healthy behaviors are emphasized and weight-related teasing and behaviors are not tolerated, students will have a greater opportunity to develop healthy body-related attitudes and behaviors. For example, through involvement in a school-based prevention program, our case study Mia would learn strategies to respect her body and care for it in healthy ways (e.g., enjoyable exercise and nourishing foods) and also learn about the dangers of dieting. Mia would also learn the importance of not comparing her body to others. Mia would learn stress management techniques to better cope with school pressures in other ways than through excessive exercise and food restriction. She would learn how the media inappropriately teaches people that they can change their lives by changing their bodies and how to combat this influence by moving towards self-acceptance. She would also learn communication and interpersonal skills to remind her that friendship is not based on the size of her body, and how to assert herself in challenging social situations. Mia would also be encouraged to engage in self-caring behaviors. As well, other students and teachers would learn to not make weight-related comments, which would reduce the social pressures Mia experiences to "be thinner." Through a school-based prevention program, Mia's school environment would evolve into one of tolerance and acceptance.

Despite prevention efforts, some individuals may slip through the cracks and develop eating disordered thoughts and behaviors. When this occurs, early identification of at-risk individuals is critical to improve the chances of successful recovery.

Early Identification

Early intervention efforts are needed to prevent the development of more serious eating disorder symptoms (Merrill, 2008; Russell & Ryder, 2001a). There is a greater chance for recovery if key others work together to combat the symptoms of the illness as early as possible (Lask & Bryant-Waugh, 1999; Mond, Hay, Rodgers, & Owen, 2008; Powers & Johnson, 1999; Vitousek et al., 1998). This process may begin with the school counselor first identifying the at-risk individual, then talking with the student and parents, and making an appropriate referral. A referral to an eating disorder specialist or treatment team is necessary, as school counselors are not likely able to provide long-term treatment. Once a student is being treated by a specialist outside of the school, the role of the school counselor becomes supporting the student in recovery at the school level.

It is difficult to identify individuals who may be at risk of developing an eating disorder because the specific behaviors associated with eating disorders (i.e., bingeing, purging, excessive exercise) are generally done in secrecy and few people reach the emaciated state associated with anorexia nervosa. Instead, as in the case study of Mia, individuals with disordered eating and symptoms of eating disorders may present as fully functional, organized, enthusiastic, and intelligent individuals involved in a wide range of activities (Vitousek et al., 1998). However, there are a number of readily observable food- and body-related behaviors, as well as social and psychological warning signs, that may signal the need for intervention. Table 4.1 presents some of the most common warning signs of eating disorders, with dieting being the most significant signal of a potential problem.

Not all behaviors and attitudes may be observed in every individual with disordered eating or body image problems; however, a combination of these behaviors and attitudes may warrant the need for further investigation. For example, our case study Mia demonstrated many food- and body-related behaviors that would be noticed by teachers and friends (e.g., dieting, fasting, vegetarianism, skipping meals, counting calories and fat grams, obsessive rumination about food, and excessive exercise). She became more isolated from friends, and hid her problems from her family. Mia's observable behaviors indicate a problem that requires further investigation.

The tremendous variety of warning signs reinforces the notion that weight and body image concerns are not "one size fits all." This indicates a need for an individualized approach to assessment and intervention.

Early Assessment

A comprehensive assessment is useful for providing direction for an intervention (Merrill, 2008). Recommended assessment protocol includes initial screening questions, self-report questionnaires and/or a structured interview, and referral to a professional for a formal assessment. School counselors may ask initial screening questions about dieting (e.g., "Mia, why do you think you need to diet?"), body image (e.g., "Mia, what makes you worry about your body size or shape?"),

T A B L E 4.1   Common Warning Signs for Eating Disorders

Food-Related Behaviors	Body-Related Behaviors	Psychological Warning Signs	Social Behaviors
Dieting (may include counting calories and fat grams, excessive use of "low fat" or "health" foods)[1,2]	Body checking behaviors[5] (e.g., weighing oneself; repeatedly, touching or pinching parts of the body that may be considered "fat" [e.g., stomach, arms, under the chin])	Complaining of "feeling fat"[9,10,11]	Avoiding social situations to avoid eating in front of others[1,2] or exercise[10]
Fasting[1,2]	Mirror-checking behaviors[5] (this may include any reflective surface)	Moodiness (e.g., depression, anxiety, irritability)[9,10,11]	Hiding behaviors from friends and family[10]
Complaining of food allergies or hypoglycaemia when there is no medical evidence[1,2]	Comparing one's body to media images[6,7]	Difficulty expressing emotions[9,10,11]	Increasing intolerance of others[10]
Skipping meals or refusing food[1,2]	Excessive exercise (e.g., solitary, while ill or injured)[8]	A critical attitude or over-sensitivity to criticism[9,10,11]	Not flexible or adaptable[10]
Vegetarian diet[1,3,4]		Perfectionist thinking[9,10,11]	
Obsessive rumination about food[1] (e.g., collecting recipes, cooking meals without eating them)		Competitiveness[9,10,11]	
		A sense of over-responsibility[9,10,11]	
		Conformity, external locus of control[9,10,11]	
		Low self-esteem[9,10,11]	
		Demonstration of "black-and-white" thinking[9,10,11]	
		Excessive concern about grades[12]	

NOTE: [1]Thompson & Sherman, 1993; [2]Kilbourne, 1999; [3]Lindeman, Stark, & Latvala, 2000; [4]Sullivan & Damani, 2000; [5]Ruffolo, Phillips, Menard, Fay, & Weisberg, 2006; [6]Thompson & Stice, 2001; [7]Brown & Dittmar, 2005; [8]Davis, 2000; [9]Kaye, Klump, Frank, & Strober, 2000; [10]Rogers & Petrie, 2001; [11]Vitousek et al., 1998; [12]Tate, 2000.

and self-esteem (e.g., "Mia, how does thinking about your weight affect how you feel about yourself?"). Self-report questionnaires and/or structured interviews are useful in identifying the presence and severity of eating-related symptoms. A wide number of well-researched and valid structured interviews and self-report questionnaires for the assessment of eating disorder symptoms have been developed (for a description of some of these items and others, see Anderson, Lavender, Milnes, & Simmons, 2009; Crowther & Sherwood, 1997; Yanover & Thompson, 2009). Even with the use of structured assessment instruments, individuals with eating disorders may not report their symptoms reliably for self-protective reasons or out of shame (Vitousek et al., 1998). Therefore, a referral for an assessment by a professional who specializes in the intervention of eating disorders is necessary. However, before an appropriate referral can be made, it is important to express one's concerns to the at-risk student and his/her parents.

TALKING ABOUT EATING DISORDERS WITH AT-RISK STUDENTS AND THEIR CAREGIVERS

People often do not know what to say when communicating their concern to an individual who presents with body image concerns or behaviors related to eating disorders. However, *not* discussing one's concerns enables the at-risk individual to continue with unhealthy behaviors that may potentially endanger the person's life (Thompson & Sherman, 1993). Denial and resistance are common when students with eating disorder behaviors are first confronted about their condition (Rogers & Petrie, 2001; Vitousek et al., 1998). For example, our case study Mia may insist that "everything is fine," "I really do need to lose weight," or "I'm just trying to get in shape." Denial and resistance are often directed against the fear of weight gain, losing control, and feelings of helplessness (Vitousek et al., 1998). Knowing that concerns will likely be met with denial and resistance should not deter school counselors from expressing their concerns and insisting on obtaining a professional's opinion.

Bock (1999) recommended the following three guidelines for approaching at-risk individuals and their parents:

1. Demonstrate support and concern for the child's health and well-being
2. Express empathy and understanding to facilitate an open communication about the problem
3. State honest, objective statements about the behaviors of concern, followed by insisting on obtaining a professional's opinion.

Non-judgmental, empathic, and truthful statements about the behaviors of concern are recommended when confronting an at-risk individual and his/her parents (Bock). For example, when speaking to an individual, the following statements may be helpful: "I'm concerned about you, Mia. You seem tense and worried, you have stopped being with your friends, and you seem sad";

"Mia, I can't keep this a secret. I've see you throwing out your lunch, and that is dangerous. We need to get you some help. Would you like me to go with you to talk to your parents, or would you prefer me to tell them first myself?"

When speaking with parents, the following statements may reflect one's concerns in an open and honest manner: "I'm concerned about your daughter's health and well-being. She is throwing out her lunches, seems overly concerned about her grades, and has stopped engaging in her usual activities. I am concerned enough to recommend seeking a consultation with a professional who specializes in problems with body image and disordered eating." It is important to note that parents may have an especially hard time understanding that such behaviors may be problematic, as they may suffer from their own need to be perfect, and/or struggle with their own body image issues. To increase the chance of a successful interaction, stick to the facts, do not offer judgment or diagnosis, and reiterate your concern about the student's health.

Making a Referral for Outside Intervention

Assuming total responsibility for the intervention of a student with an eating disorder is beyond the normal responsibilities of school counselors. Therefore, working with the family to make a referral for assessment and intervention is essential (Russell & Ryder, 2001b). A specialized intervention team including the family physician, a nutritionist, a mental health therapist, and a family therapist is necessary in order to address the multi-faceted nature of an eating disorder. Together, the intervention team makes decisions about assessment, intervention options, and when to involve the family and school staff (if necessary). A professional school counselor can be an important member of the intervention team by helping provide support to the recovering student at the school and acting as a liaison between the various involved individuals (e.g., school administration, other mental health care providers and physicians). School counselors will also want to ensure that they liaise effectively with teachers to address needed academic accommodations. Depending on the unique issues of the student involved, school counselors may also have a role to play as liaison to the student's peers to aid in the maintenance of positive relationships. Acting as a liaison between the specialized intervention team and the school is the fundamental role for school counselors.

Supporting the Student in Recovery

Recovery from an eating disorder is an ongoing process of balancing and rebalancing the self, even once unhealthy behaviors are diminished and the body is stabilized (Garrett, 1997; Pike, 1998; Reindl, 2001). The primary focus of intervention for eating disorders is to restore the individual to a more normalized, moderate, and functional lifestyle while addressing the extremes of attitudes and behaviors. Intervention teams may integrate a variety of approaches to intervention based on each individual's specific needs, the age of onset, severity, and longevity of the eating disorder.

Phases of Intervention

It is generally accepted that the intervention of eating disorders occurs in three phases: (1) a medical approach focuses on the restoration of a healthy weight and/or normalization of eating behaviors, (2) a psychological/social/familial approach focuses on changing attitudes and behaviors, and (3) relapse prevention (Garner, Vitousek, & Pike, 1997; Vitousek et al., 1998; Wilson, Fairburn, & Agras, 1997). These phases may not necessarily proceed in a linear manner due to the cyclical nature of eating disorder recovery.

1. Medical Focus   The first phase in the intervention for eating disorders focuses on the stabilization of weight and normalization of eating and exercise habits (Garner et al., 1997; Vitousek et al., 1998). Hospitalization and specialized medical intervention may be necessary if the individual demonstrates severe malnourishment and an inability to engage in intervention on an outpatient basis. At this phase, the responsibilities of the school counselor would be to act as the liaison to the school and provide support by reinforcing the intervention goals. Helping the student plan manageable course loads in consultation with the intervention team would also be an asset, as a student's health and well-being overrides academic achievement. In our case study, Mia would not be hospitalized at this stage because her behaviors have not become life-threatening. However, should Mia ever require hospitalization, it may be necessary for the school counselor to work with her to adapt her academic course load according to the recommendations of the treatment team. As well, she will likely need continued reassurance that her grades and future academic goals will not suffer while she is beginning the road to wellness.

2. Psychological Focus   The second phase generally evolves once the body becomes stabilized, and other issues take precedence over physical concerns. Specific interventions may include cognitive restructuring (e.g., identifying and specifying problem thoughts), teaching problem solving skills and new coping strategies, and helping to develop appropriate emotional expression (Garner et al., 1997; Wilson et al., 1997). It is also important to address shape and weight concerns, develop strategies to improve self-esteem and body image, and address concerns with perfectionism (Garner et al.; Wilson et al.). Family conflicts and interpersonal functioning may also need to be addressed by the school counselor and/or other professionals (Garner et al.; Wilson et al.). Self-monitoring can help individuals regain a sense of control over their thoughts and behaviors and transform unhealthy food and exercise behaviors into health-enhancing behaviors (Crowther & Sherwood, 1997; Garner et al.; Tantillo, 2000; Wilson et al.). At this stage, school counselors may provide support to students by assisting them in considering alternative points of view, other than the black-and-white thinking that often accompanies eating-disordered thinking (Wilson et al.).

Many students at this stage of recovery may be overly concerned with their school achievement. In collaboration with the intervention team, school counselors may assist with self-monitoring in order to develop and maintain a balance between work and relaxation, as well as develop short-term, realistic academic goals. For some students, it may be important to encourage them to reduce their workload in order to help them focus on developing more balance in their lives. Support at the school level is important at this stage to help prevent overly conscientious students from falling back into old thinking and behavior patterns that may contribute to recurring eating disorder attitudes and behaviors. In our case study, Mia would likely benefit from cognitive restructuring around the need to exercise versus the need to socialize, and the negative belief that other people may not like her because of her body size. The development of a daily schedule that includes a balance of school, socializing, and relaxation would benefit Mia as she begins to adapt to more positive attitudes and behaviors.

3. Relapse Prevention   The third phase of eating disorder intervention involves the development of relapse prevention strategies (Garner et al., 1997; Keel, Dorer, Franko, Jackson, & Herzog, 2005; Reindl, 2001; Wilson et al., 1997). Unfortunately, relapse is common in individuals with eating disorders, even up to 12 years after recovery (Schneider & Irons, 1997; Keel et al.). Maisel, Epston, and Borden (2004) called the return of eating disorder symptoms a "comeback," during which an individual may resort to previous unhealthy behaviors during times of stress. Individuals with eating disorders may continue to be vulnerable to body preoccupation and dissatisfaction, drive for thinness, obsessive thoughts and behaviors, emotional restraint, unusual eating habits, perfectionism, and negative affect (Kaye et al., 2000; Pike, 1998; Reindl, 2001). Relapse prevention includes both anticipating future difficulties, especially during potentially stressful circumstances (e.g., final exams, graduation, preparation for university or work), and the development of self-care strategies for combating the return of eating disorder symptoms. School counselors may contribute to maintenance and relapse prevention plans by helping students prepare for inevitable challenges related to school, exploring an individual's stress triggers, and encouraging them to develop rational and healthy coping plans and future goals. Although our case study, Mia, may make positive gains in developing a more positive body image, unforeseen stressors may trigger a comeback of familiar attitudes and behaviors. When such situations arise, school counselors may be able to use supportive intervention approaches to assist students in preventing relapse.

SUPPORTIVE INTERVENTION APPROACHES
FOR SCHOOL COUNSELORS

Although there are a number of researched interventions for eating disorders (see Bardick et al., 2004; Keel & Haedt, 2008; or Sperry, Roehrig, & Thompson, 2009, for a comprehensive listing), well-established interventions for school counselors remain sparse. Overall, we recommend that school counselors implement interventions and supportive strategies as suggested by the intervention team in order to effectively meet the recovery needs of the student at the school level. For example, some students may require individual counseling, while other students may require assistance with planning a lighter course load or making up for classes missed if they have been in an in-patient intervention setting. Specific interventions appropriate for school counselors to use with individuals recovering from eating disorders and body image concerns include cognitive-behavioral therapy (CBT), guided imagery, and narrative therapy.

Cognitive-Behavioral Therapy

CBT is a widely researched, effective intervention for eating disorders (Cooper & Shafran, 2008; Garner et al., 1997; Keel & Haedt, 2008; Schumann & Hickner, 2009; Sysko & Hildebrandt, 2009; Williamson & Netemeyer, 2000; Wilson et al., 1997). CBT encourages an examination of the contradictions in thought and behavior that occur with eating disorders, specific purposes of eating disorder symptoms (e.g., bingeing as a response to stress), advantages and disadvantages of certain beliefs and behaviors, as well as the costs and benefits of change (Vitousek et al., 1998). For the school counselor, the use of CBT may help students examine their thoughts about behaviors that happen at school, such as eating lunch or snacks with other students present, appropriately balancing school work with recreation, and examining their beliefs about achievement and success in their future goals and plans. It is also important to discuss with students the challenges in not dieting and trying to lose weight when other students and teachers are very likely engaging in and discussing those very behaviors.

Guided Imagery

Guided imagery is sometimes used in clinical settings (Paley & Rabinor, 2000), and if used correctly and carefully in school settings, may be another appropriate and constructive intervention technique for school counselors. The use of guided imagery is a respectful and non-intrusive intervention that may help individuals experience relaxation, reduce anxiety, and imagine different outcomes for stressful situations. Relaxation through guided imagery can be healing, and guided imagery may be helpful to shape reality (Hutchinson, 1994). Guided imagery that uses the specific needs of the student to guide the focus of the intervention can be very helpful.

Narrative Therapy

Widely used in clinical settings, narrative therapy, or the retelling and rewriting of personal narratives as therapeutic process, may also be a useful intervention for school counselors in addressing eating disorders (Garrett, 1997; Lock, Epston, & Maisel, 2004; Reindl, 2001; Russell, 2000). Through the use of narrative therapy, school counselors encourage individuals to begin imagining a positive outcome to their personal story of recovery. A narrative approach may also be used for goal setting, as individuals first imagine the life story they would like to have, and then

T A B L E 4.2   **Helpful Web Sites Addressing Eating Disorders**

Organization	Web Site
Academy of Eating Disorders	http://www.aedweb.org/eating_disorders/prevalence.cfm
Alliance for Eating Disorder Awareness (The Alliance)	http://www.eatingdisorderinfo.org/
Healthy Weight Network	http://www.healthyweightnetwork.com/
National Association for Anorexia Nervosa and Associated Eating Disorders	http://www.anad.org/
National Eating Disorders Association	http://www.nationaleatingdisorders.org/
National Eating Disorder Information Center	http://www.nedic.ca/
National Institute of Mental Health	http://www.nimh.nih.gov/health/publications/eating-disorders/complete-index.shtml
Something Fishy: Website on Eating Disorders	http://www.something-fishy.org/

set goals to achieve the desired outcome. Showing videos and/or reading about other people's stories of recovery may also be helpful.

School counselors can utilize their role as the liaison between the specialized intervention team and the school to support students with eating disorders through CBT strategies, guided imagery, and narrative approaches and draw upon their unique knowledge of the school environment to support the student in the school setting. For additional ideas, one can consult numerous relevant Web sites (see Table 4.2).

SUMMARY

School counselors play an important role in both the prevention and identification of eating disorders and in supporting students during the recovery process. The recommendations in this chapter are designed to provide school counselors with an awareness of how to identify at-risk students, implement school-based prevention programs, make appropriate referrals, and support recovering students at the school level. Prevention and intervention efforts implemented by school counselors may be helpful in improving students' body images; encouraging school-age children and adolescents to question beliefs about "thin" and "fat"; developing healthy and active lifestyles; and demonstrating tolerance and respect for people with bodies of all shapes, sizes, and physical abilities.

REFERENCES

Academy of Eating Disorders. (n.d.). *Prevalence of eating disorders*. Retrieved May 30, 2009, from http://www.aedweb.org/eating_disorders/prevalence.cfm

Akos, P., & Levitt, D. H. (2002). Promoting healthy body image in middle school. *Professional School Counseling, 6,* 138–144.

American Psychiatric Association. (2000a). *Diagnostic and statistical manual of mental disorders* (4th ed., Text Revision). Washington, DC: Author.

American Psychiatric Association. (2000b). Practice guideline for the treatment of patients with eating disorders (revision). *American Journal of Psychiatry, 157,* 1–38.

Anderson, D. A., Lavender, J. M. Milnes, S. M., & Simmons, A. M. (2009). Assessment of eating disturbances in children and adolescents. In L. Smolak & J. K. Thompson (Eds.), *Body image, eating disorders, and obesity in youth: Assessment, prevention, and treatment* (2nd ed., pp. 193–214). Washington, DC: American Psychological Association.

Austin, S. B., Field, A. E., Wiecha, J., Peterson, K. E., & Gortmaker, S. (2005). The impact of a school-based obesity prevention trial on disordered weight-control behaviors in early adolescent girls. *Archive of Pediatric Adolescent Medicine, 159,* 225–230.

Bardick, A. D., Bernes, K. B., McCulloch, A. R. M., Witko, K. D., Spriddle, J. W., & Roest, A. R. (2004). Eating disorder intervention, prevention, and treatment: Recommendations for school counselors. *Professional School Counseling, 8,* 168–175.

Boisseau, C. L., Thompson-Brenner, H., Eddy, K. T., & Satir, D. A. (2009). Impulsivity and personality variables in adolescents with eating disorders. *The Journal of Nervous and Mental Disease, 197,* 251–259.

Bock, L. P. (1999). Secrets and denial: The costs of not getting help. In R. Lemberg & L. Cohn (Eds.), *Eating disorders: A reference sourcebook* (pp. 43–44). Phoenix, AR: Oryx Press.

Body Image Works. (2005) *Body Image Kits*. Retrieved June 1, 2009, from www.bodyimageworks.com

Brown, A., & Dittmar, H. (2005). Think "thin" and feel bad: The role of appearance motivated schema activation, attention level, and thin-ideal internalization for young women's responses to ultra-thin media ideals. *Journal of Social and Clinical Psychology, 24,* 1088–1113.

Butryn, M. L., & Wadden, T. A. (2005). Treatment of overweight in children and adolescents: Does dieting increase the risk of eating disorders? *International Journal of Eating Disorders, 37,* 285–293.

Cavanaugh, C. J., & Lemberg, R. (1999). What we know about eating disorders: Facts and statistics. In R. Lemberg & L. Cohn (Eds.), *Eating disorders: A reference sourcebook* (pp. 7–12). Phoenix, AZ: Oryx Press.

Choate, L. H. (2005). Toward a theoretical model of women's body image resilience. *Journal of Counseling & Development, 83,* 320–330.

Choate, L. H. (2007). Counseling adolescent girls for body image resilience: Strategies for school counselors. *Professional School Counseling, 10,* 317–326.

Cooper, Z., & Shafran, R. (2008). Cognitive behaviour therapy for eating disorders. *Behavioural & Cognitive Psychotherapy, 36,* 713–722.

Crandall, C. S. (1994). Prejudice against fat people: Ideology and self-interest. *Journal of Personality and Social Psychology, 66*, 882–895.

Crandall, C. S., D'Anello, S. D., Sakalli, N., Wieczorkowski, G., & Feather, N. T. (2001). An Attribution-value model of prejudice: Anti-fat attitudes in six nations. *Personal and Social Psychology Bulletin, 27*, 30–37.

Crowther, J. H., & Sherwood, N. E. (1997). Assessment. In D. Garner & P. Garfinkel (Eds.), *Handbook of treatment for eating disorders* (2nd ed., pp. 34–49). New York: Guilford.

Davis, C. (2000). Exercise abuse. *International Journal of Sport Psychology, 31*, 278–289.

Dohnt, H. K., & Tiggemann, M. (2008). Promoting positive body image in young girls: An evaluation of 'Shapesville'. *European Eating Disorders Review: The Journal of Eating Disorders, 16*, 222–233.

Garner, D. M., Vitousek, K. M., & Pike, K. M. (1997). Cognitive-behavioral therapy for anorexia nervosa. In D. Garner & P. Garfinkel (Eds.), *Handbook of treatment for eating disorders* (2nd ed., pp. 94–144). New York: Guilford.

Garrett, C. J. (1997). Recovery from anorexia nervosa: A sociological perspective. *International Journal of Eating Disorders, 21*, 261–272.

Graber, J., Archibald, A., & Brooks-Gunn, J. (1999). The role of parents in the emergence, maintenance and prevention of eating problems and disorders. In N. Piran, M. Levine, & C. Steiner-Adair (Eds.), *Preventing eating disorders* (pp. 44–62). Philadelphia, PA: Taylor & Francis.

Gregorio, L. (2009). STAR program. *Eating Disorders, 17*, 183–184.

Haines, J., Neumark-Sztainer, D., Perry, C. L., Hannan, P. J., & Levine, M. P. (2006). V. I. K. (Very Important Kids): A school-based program designed to reduce teasing and unhealthy weight-control behaviors. *Health Education Research, 21*, 884–895.

Haines, J., Neumark-Sztainer, D., Thiel, L. (2007). Addressing weight-related issues in an elementary school: What do students, parents, and school staff recommend? *Eating Disorders, 15*, 5–21.

Hutchinson, M. G. (1994). Imagining ourselves whole: A feminist approach to treating body image disorders. In P. Fallon, M. Katzman, & S. Wooley (Eds.), *Feminist perspectives on eating disorders* (pp. 152–168). New York: Guilford.

Jensen, B. (2009, May 28). Childhood obesity reaching critical levels quickly. *The Daily News Online*. Retrieved June 1, 2009, from http://www.richmond-dailynews.com/news.php?id=3170

Kaye, W. H., Klump, K. L., Frank, G. K. W., & Strober, M. (2000). Anorexia and bulimia nervosa. *Annual Reviews of Medicine, 51*, 299–313.

Keel, P. K., Dorer, D. J., Franko, D. L., Jackson, S. C., & Herzog, D. B. (2005). Postremission predictors of relapse in women with eating disorders. *American Journal of Psychiatry, 162*, 2263–2268.

Keel, P. K., & Haedt, A. (2008). Evidence-based psychosocial treatments for eating problems and eating disorders. *Journal of Clinical Child & Adolescent Psychology, 37*, 39–61.

Klaczynski, P. A., Goold, K. W., & Mudry, J. J. (2004). Culture, obesity stereotypes, self-esteem, and the "thin ideal": A social identity perspective. *Journal of Youth and Adolescence, 33*, 307–317.

Kostanski, M., & Gullone, E. (2007). The impact of teasing on children's body image. *Journal of Child & Family Studies, 16,* 307–319.

Lask, B., & Bryant-Waugh, R. (1999). Prepubertal eating disorders. In N. Piran, M. Levine, & C. Steiner-Adair (Eds.), *Preventing eating disorders* (pp. 476–483). Philadelphia, PA: Taylor & Francis.

Levine, M., Piran, N., & Stoddard, C. (1999). Mission more probable: Media literacy, activism, and advocacy as primary prevention. In N. Piran, M. Levine, & C. Steiner-Adair (Eds.), *Preventing eating disorders* (pp. 1–25). Philadelphia, PA: Taylor & Francis.

Levitt, D. H. (2003). Drive for thinness and fear of fat: Separate yet related constructs? *Eating Disorders, 11,* 21–234.

Lindeman, M., Stark, K., & Latvala, K. (2000). Vegetarianism and eating-disordered thinking. *Eating Disorders, 8,* 157–165.

Lock, A., Epston, E., & Maisel, R. (2004). Countering that which is called anorexia. *Narrative Inquiry, 14,* 275–301

Lock, J., & Jaffee, L. (1996). *The bodywise woman* (2nd ed.). Champaign, IL: Human Kinetics.

Maisel, R., Epston, D., & Borden, A. (2004). *Biting the hand that starves you: Inspiring resistance to anorexia/bulimia.* New York: W.W. Norton.

McVey, G., Gusella, J., Tweed, S., & Ferrari, M. (2009). A controlled evaluation of web-based training for teachers and public health practitioners on the prevention of eating disorders. *Eating Disorders, 17,* 1–26.

McVey, G., Tweed, S., & Blackmore, E. (2007). Healthy Schools—Healthy Kids: A controlled evaluation of a comprehensive universal eating disorder prevention program. *Body Image, 4,* 115–136.

Merrill, K. M. (2008). *Behavioral, social, and emotional assessment of children and adolescents* (3rd ed.). New York: Lawrence Erlbaum.

Mond, J. M., Hay, P., Rodgers, B., & Owen, C. (2008). Mental health literacy and eating disorders: What do women with bulimic eating disorders think and know about bulimia nervosa and its treatment? *Journal of Mental Health, 17,* 565–575.

Monro, F., & Huon, G. (2005). Media–portrayed idealized images, body shame, and appearance anxiety. *International Journal of Eating Disorders, 38,* 85–90.

National Association of State Boards of Education, & Pekruhn, C. (2009). *Preventing childhood obesity: A school health policy guide.* Retrieved June 1, 2009, from http://www.rwjf.org/childhoodobesity/product.jsp?id=42472

Neumark–Sztainer, D., Levine, M. P., Paxton, S. J., Smolak, L., Pirna, N., & Wertheim, E. H. (2006). Prevention of body dissatisfaction and disordered eating: What's next? *Eating Disorders, 14,* 265–286.

Paley, V., & Rabinor, J. R. (2000). Hatching a new identity: Transforming the anorexic patient and the therapist. *Eating Disorders, 8,* 67–76.

Pike, K. M. (1998). Long-term course of anorexia nervosa: Response, relapse, remission, and recovery. *Clinical Psychology Review, 18,* 447–475.

Pope, H. G., Jr., Phillips, K. A., & Olivardia, R. (2000). *The Adonis complex: How to identify, treat, and prevent body obsession in men and boys.* New York: Touchstone.

Powers, P., & Johnson, C. (1999). Small victories: Prevention of eating disorders among elite athletes. In N. Piran, M. Levine, & C. Steiner-Adair (Eds.), *Preventing eating disorders* (pp. 241–254). Philadelphia, PA: Taylor & Francis.

Reindl, S. (2001). *Sensing the self: Women's recovery from bulimia.* Cambridge, MA: Harvard University Press.

Roehrig, M., Thompson, J. K, Brannick, M., & van den Berg, P. (2006). Dissonance-based eating disorder prevention program: A preliminary dismantling investigation. *International Journal of Eating Disorders, 39,* 1–10.

Rogers, R. L., & Petrie, T. A. (2001). Psychological correlates of anorexia and bulimic symptomology. *Journal of Counseling & Development, 79,* 178–186.

Ruffolo, J. S., Phillips, K. A., Mendard, W., Fay, C., & Weisberg, R. A. (2006). Comorbidity of body dysmorphic disorder and eating disorders: Severity of psychopathology and body image disturbance. *International Journal of Eating Disorders, 39,* 11–19.

Russell, S. (2000). A narrative approach to treating eating disorders: A case study. *Guidance and Counselling, 15*(4), 10–13.

Russell, S., & Ryder, S. (2001a). BRIDGE (Building the relationship between body image and disordered eating graph and explanation): A tool for parents and professionals. *Eating Disorders: The Journal of Treatment and Prevention, 9,* 1–14.

Russell, S., & Ryder, S. (2001b). BRIDGE 2 (Building the relationship between body image and disordered eating graph and explanation): Interventions and transitions. *Eating Disorders: The Journal of Treatment and Prevention, 9,* 15–27.

Russell-Mayhew, S. (2006). The last word: stop the war on weight: obesity and eating disorder prevention working together toward health. *Eating Disorders, 14,* 253–263

Russell-Mayhew, S. (2007). Preventing a continuum of disordered eating: Going beyond the individual. *The Prevention Researcher, 14,* 7–10.

Russell-Mayhew, S., Arthur, N., & Ewashen, C. (2007). Targeting students, teachers and parents in a wellness-based prevention program in schools. *Eating Disorders, 15,* 159–181.

Russell-Mayhew, S., Arthur, N., & Ewashen, C. (in press). Community capacity building in schools: Parent and teacher reflections from an eating disorder program. *Alberta Journal of Educational Research.*

Schneider, J., & Irons, R. (1997). Treatment of gambling, eating, and sex addictions. In N. Miller, M. Gold, & D. Smith (Eds.), *Manual of Therapeutics for Addictions* (pp. 225–245). New York: Wiley-Liss.

Schumann, S-A. & Hickner, J. (2009). Suspect an eating disorder? Suggest CBT. *Journal of Family Practice, 58,* 265–266.

Smolak, L. (1999). Elementary school curricula for the primary prevention of eating problems. In N. Piran, M. Levine, & C. Steiner-Adair (Eds.), *Preventing eating disorders* (pp. 85–104). Philadelphia, PA: Taylor & Francis.

Smolak, L., Harris, B., Levine, M., & Shisslak, C. (2001). Teachers: The forgotten influence on the success of prevention programs. *Eating Disorders: The Journal of Treatment and Prevention, 9,* 261–265.

Smolak, L., & Thompson, J. K. (Eds.). (2008). Body image, eating disorders, and obesity in youth: Assessment, prevention, and treatment (2nd ed.). Washington, DC: American Psychological Association.

Sperry, S., Roehrig, M., & Thompson, J. K. (2009). Treatment of eating disorders in childhood and adolescence. In L. Smolak & J. K. Thompson (Eds.), *Body image, eating disorders, and obesity in youth: Assessment, prevention, and treatment* (2nd ed., pp. 261–280). Washington, DC: American Psychological Association.

Steiner-Adair, C. (1994). The politics of prevention. In P. Fallon, M. Katzman, & S. Wooley (Eds.), *Feminist perspectives on eating disorders* (pp. 381–394). New York: Guilford.

Steinhausen, H. C. (2009). Outcome of eating disorders. *Child and Adolescent Psychiatric Clinics of North America, 18*, 225–242.

Sullivan, V., & Damani, S. (2000). Vegetarianism and eating disorders: Partners in crime? *European Eating Disorders Review, 8*, 263–266

Sweetingham, R., & Waller, G. (2008). Childhood experiences of being bullied and teased in the eating disorders. *European Eating Disorders Review, 16*, 401–407.

Sysko, R., & Hildebrandt, T. (2009). Cognitive-behavioural therapy for individuals with bulimia nervosa and a co-occurring substance use disorder. *European Eating Disorders Review, 17*, 89–100.

Tantillo, M. (2000). Short-term relational group therapy for women with bulimia nervosa. *Eating Disorders: The Journal of Treatment and Prevention, 8*, 99–121.

Tate, A. (2000). Schooling. In B. Lask & R. Bryant-Waugh (Eds), *Anorexia nervosa and related eating disorders in childhood and adolescence* (2nd ed., pp. 323–247). Hove, East Sussex, UK: Psychology Press.

Thomas, J. J., Vartanian, L. R., & Brownell, K. D. (2009). The relationship Between Eating Disorder Not Otherwise Specified (EDNOS) and officially recognized eating disorders: Meta-analysis and implications for DSM. *Psychological Bulletin, 135*, 407–433.

Thompson, R. A., & Sherman, R. T. (1993). *Helping athletes with eating disorders.* Champaign, IL: Human Kinetics.

Thompson, J. K., & Stice, E. (2001). Thin-ideal internalization: Mounting evidence for a new risk factor for body-image disturbance and eating pathology. *Current Directions in Psychological Science, 10*, 181–183.

Varnado-Sullivan, P. J., & Horton, R. A. (2006). Acceptability of programs for the prevention of eating disorders. *Journal of Clinical Psychology, 62*, 687–703.

Varnado-Sullivan, P. J., Zucker, N., Williamson, D. A., Reas, D., Thaw, J., & Netemeyer, S. B. (2001). Development and implementation of the Body Logic Program for adolescents: A two-stage prevention program for eating disorders. *Cognitive and Behavioral Practice, 8*, 248–259.

Vitousek, K., Watson, S., & Wilson, G. (1998). Enhancing motivation for change in treatment resistant eating disorders. *Clinical Psychology Review, 18*, 391–420.

Williamson, D., & Netemeyer, S. (2000). Cognitive-behavior therapy. In K. Miller & S. Mizes (Eds.), *Comparative treatments for eating disorders* (pp. 61–81). New York: Springer.

Wilson, G. T., Fairburn, C. G., & Agras, W. S. (1997). Cognitive-behavioral therapy for bulimia nervosa. In D. Garner & P. Garfinkel (Eds.), *Handbook of treatment for eating disorders* (2nd ed., pp. 67–93). New York: Guilford.

Yager, J., & Powers, P. (Eds.). (2007). *Clinical manual of eating disorders.* Washington, DC: American Psychiatric Publishing.

Yanover, T., & Thompson, J. K. (2009). Assessment of body image in children and adolescents. In L. Smolak & J. K. Thompson (Eds.), *Body image, eating disorders, and obesity in youth: Assessment, prevention, and treatment* (2nd ed., pp. 177–192). Washington, DC: American Psychological Association.

Chapter 5

Substance Abuse

Implications for School Counseling Practice

GLENN W. LAMBIE

University of Central Florida

Substance abuse-related problems are prevalent in school-age children and pose a significant danger for students, possibly resulting in serious psychological, social, educational, vocational, and legal consequences. In schools, substance abuse-related issues tend to manifest in the family system (parental/caregiver substance abuse, children of alcoholics) at the elementary, middle, and secondary levels; while substance abuse by students generally begins during middle and high school. This chapter introduces an array of substance abuse related issues professional school counselors frequently encounter. Additionally, definitions, prognosis, observable warning signs, symptoms, and school-based intervention strategies are presented. We begin with two real-world case studies to frame the subsequent discussion.

Samantha: An Elementary School–Based Case Study

While providing elementary school–based counseling services, a counselor received a referral for a 9-year-old Grade 4 student named Samantha. Samantha had been referred to the school counselor by her teacher, who was concerned because Samantha was often inattentive and was not doing well in her class. The teacher also reported that Samantha often appeared to be tired (e.g., would sleep in class) and moody, her grades fluctuated, and she was frequently absent. Further, the teacher explained that she had tried to contact Samantha's parents, but had not heard back from them.

When the school counselor first met with Samantha, she appeared quiet and polite, but did not seem comfortable talking. When asked if she liked to draw, she replied, "Yes, I do like to draw; I am artistic." The counselor asked if Samantha would draw a picture of her family doing an activity together. Samantha asked, "Can I include my dog?" The counselor said she could, and passed her some paper, canyons, colored pencils, and markers. As Samantha began to draw, she appeared more comfortable and talkative. Once she had completed her picture of her family,

---

Jeff: A High School–Based Case Study

A professional school counselor worked in a high school and was a team member of the school's Student Assistance Program. A Student Assistance Program is a school-based comprehensive prevention, intervention, and support services program for students, employing a systemic team approach that is designed to support students exhibiting risk behaviors impeding their educational achievement. During this time, a 16-year-old student named Jeff was referred to the counselor for academic and behavioral problems. Jeff was an intelligent and social student, as was evident in his high standardized achievement assessment scores and in observed interactions with his peers. Additionally, teachers reported that while Jeff had at first been friendly and gregarious, over the past few months he had become increasingly moody and uncooperative in completing school assignments. When the counselor first met with Jeff, he was polite and open to talking. As the counselor inquired about Jeff's academic problems, he acknowledged that his grades had dropped over the last year upon entering high school, but it was "no big deal." Jeff further added that one of the reasons his grades were so poor during his freshman year was his suspension from school for 10 days because he was caught

---

As is evident in these two case studies, substance abuse-related issues can impact students at all levels and are common. Professional school counselors play a primary role in supporting, intervening with, and assisting these students and their families. The following section presents essential characteristics and descriptors of students with a substance abuse problem themselves, and students who may be children of alcoholics.

the counselor asked Samantha if she would explain her picture, which she promptly did. Interestingly, Samantha had drawn herself, her mother, her siblings, and the dog playing together in their home, while her father was outside talking to two other individuals. When asked who the men were who were speaking with her father, Samantha replied, "His friends; he likes to hang out with them. They hang out together and go to the races and stuff." The counselor continued to meet with Samantha and contacted her mother (after numerous unsuccessful attempts) in order to schedule a meeting with the two of them. During the meeting, Samantha's mother, Jane, explained that she was concerned about Samantha and apologized for not getting in contact with the counselor earlier. After some time, it became evident that Samantha's father may have a drinking problem, and was often not home because he was out with his friends. At this point, the counselor decided to refer Samantha to the school's children of alcoholics group, which was facilitated by a prevention specialist for the county.

with cigarettes on school grounds. He further explained that his parents were aware that he smoked, so he did not understand why the school had to suspend him when his parents were fine with it.

Following the meeting with Jeff, the school counselor referred him to the school's Student Assistance Program team. After presenting Jeff's case to the team, they decided to schedule a meeting with both Jeff and his parents. At the meeting, Jeff was present and sat between his father, John, and mother, Lisa, who had been divorced for six years. Lisa expressed concern for Jeff and his poor choices; while John expressed that Jeff was fine and it was "not that big a deal." Further, John shared with the team that he drank and smoked in high school and he had turned out fine. Throughout the meeting, Lisa and the team members expressed concern for Jeff, but John continued to maintain that Jeff would be fine. At the conclusion of the meeting, Jeff explained that he agreed with his father. He was fine and would improve his grades. However, the Student Assistance Program team concluded that Jeff was exhibiting behaviors indicative of potential substance abuse and further school-based intervention and supports services were needed.

CHARACTERISTICS AND WARNING SIGNS OF SUBSTANCE ABUSE BY STUDENTS AND IN FAMILIES

For the purposes of this chapter, *substance abuse* will be used to encompass student substance abuse, dependence, and addiction. The diagnostic criteria of adolescent substance abuse are diverse, and the behaviorally observed assessment cues are subjective (Lambie & Rokutani, 2002). According to Deas, Roberts, and Grindlinger (2005), most adolescent substance abuse assessment is based on the *Diagnostic and Statistical Manual of Mental Disorders* (DSM–IV–TR; American Psychiatric Association, 2000); however, this approach is limited because the DSM–IV–TR criterion for substance abuse was intended for adults. Additionally, it is important to note that most professional school counselors do not have the credentials and training to diagnose substance abuse; however, they must be knowledgeable about the potential warning signs of substance abuse among students so they can intervene as early as possible to provide the best interventions and support.

Student substance abuse is a pervasive problem (see Brooks & McHenry, 2009, for details). The age of first substance use has been found to significantly correlate to later substance abuse. In fact, students who begin drinking alcohol prior to age 15 are four times more likely to develop alcohol dependence than those who begin drinking at age 21. Unfortunately, the average age of first alcohol use is age 12 (Kinney, 2008).

Prevalence

Substance abuse among adolescents is pervasive, but has fortunately been in a decline in recent years (Johnston, O'Malley, Bachman, & Schulenberg, 2006). Even with this decline, the statistics for substance abuse among school-age children are alarming. According to Substance Abuse and Mental Health Services Administration (SAMHSA, 2008), in 2007, 9.5% of 12- to 17-year-olds were illicit drug users. Alcohol abuse is even more prevalent. In 2007, 27.9% of youth between the ages of 12 to 20 reported having used alcohol in the previous month, and approximately 7.2 million (18.6%) of these young people were binge drinkers, while 2.3 million (6.0%) were heavy drinkers (SAMHSA). Further, the National Survey on Drug Use and Health (NSDUH, 2008) reported that many youth with substance abuse problems do not receive treatment. In 2003–2004, 6.1% of 12- to 17-year-olds exhibited symptoms necessitating treatment for alcohol abuse, and 5.4% for illicit drug use. Regarding student academic achievement, research identified a negative correlation between substance use and academic achievement, where increased substance use relates to significantly lower grades (NSDUH, 2006).

An often unacknowledged substance abuse-related issue influencing student development and achievement is alcohol abuse among parents and caregivers. Regarding its prevalence, NSDUH (2009a) reported that combined data from 2002 and 2007 indicated that approximately 12% of children younger than age 18 "lived with at least one parent who was dependent on or abused alcohol or an illicit drug during the past year" (p. 105). Additionally, research suggests that one in four school-age children resides in a home where there is alcohol abuse and dependence (Grant, 2000). These numbers may actually be conservative, as families with alcohol abuse problems are typically closed systems, contributing to underreporting and under-identification. Further, Lambie and Sias (2005) estimate that an average professional school counselor's caseload is around 477 students, approximately 120 of whom would likely be exposed to familial alcohol abuse and/or dependence. The family dysfunctionality that children of alcoholics experience often impairs these students' academic, psychological, and social development.

Potential Consequences

Student substance abuse may result in significant negative consequences including, but not limited to: poor academic achievement; the development of an addiction; incarceration; and even death. The abuse of substances during adolescence may impair a student's healthy cognitive, physical, social-emotional, and psychological development (Lambie & Smith, 2004). Substance abuse among school-age youth has been positively correlated to teenage pregnancy; anxiety and depressive disorders (internalizing behaviors; see Chapter 3); poor school performance; personal-social impairment; suicide; school attrition; truancy and absenteeism; and grade-level retention (Brook, Saar, Zhang, & Brook, 2009; Eaton, Brener, & Kann, 2007; Kinney, 2008; Lambie & Smith, 2004). The potential consequences of substance abuse can have a profound effect on students' holistic development. Readers interested in the latest study reviewing the long-term outcomes of substance abuse are encouraged to peruse Palmer et al. (2009).

Warning Signs and Identification

Student substance abuse is a complex interaction of multiple factors such as family structure and relationships, school success, peers, community, genetics, and psychological well-being. For professional school counselors to support and intervene in cases involving student substance abuse, they must have a knowledge base of its warning signs. It is important to note that some cues may be strong indictors of substance abuse; however, the presence of one symptom does not necessarily indicate that a student is abusing substances. Therefore, if school counselors observe potential symptoms of substance abuse, they should communicate their perceptions to the student and receive clarification concerning their interpretations before proceeding (Lambie & Sias, 2005).

For example, school counselors may observe students exhibiting patterns of inconsistent academic performance, absenteeism, and moodiness. If these behaviors are atypical for the student, counselors may be warranted in approaching the student about their observations. First, counselors may simply identify their perceptions concerning the changes in behavior. Next, counselors may ask an open-ended question eliciting the student to discuss his or her current life situation (e.g., How are things going for you?). Nevertheless, having an awareness and appreciation of the symptomology of substance abuse is necessary in supporting students. In addition to recognizing symptoms, it is also useful to identify antecedent risk factors in order to effectively direct students in need to available services.

The literature identifies numerous factors that may be related to student substance abuse. However, these potential indicators may be signs of other kinds of difficulties. Nevertheless, an understanding of substance abuse symptoms is vital in intervening as early as possible for the student's benefit. The warning signs of student substance abuse presented in Table 5.1 are organized by family characteristics, psychological cues, and educational indicators. These observable potential indicators are intended to provide introductory information for school counselors, enabling them to intervene appropriately in cases of *suspected* substance abuse.

T A B L E 5.1   Warning Signs of Student Substance Abuse

Areas	Potential Indicators
Familial Characteristics	Poor family communication and relationships Family history of substance abuse Being raised in a single-parent or blended family Family aggression and violence Family history of psychiatric disorders and suicide or suicide attempts Inappropriate family structure and boundaries Poor family nurturance (i.e., not emotionally warm and accepting) Absence of parent/caregiver supervision Access to alcohol and other drugs Early cigarette use Lack of rules for the young person A history of abuse and/or neglect Family appears to have little interest in school and school-related activities (e.g., sports, clubs, and parent–teacher–school counselor conferences)
Psychological Cues	Risk-taking behaviors Absence of religion/religiosity/spirituality Low self-esteem Aggressive behavior such as fighting, verbal abuse, and defiance Engaging in health-compromising behaviors Isolationism and social withdrawal Being less socially inhibited Appearing older than one's peers Rebelliousness and nonconformity Failure to form close interpersonal relationships Poor coping skills The presence of a psychological disorder, especially depression, anxiety disorders and Attention Deficit Hyperactivity Disorder (ADHD)
Educational Indicators	Low academic motivation Deterioration in academic performance Increased absenteeism and truancy School disciplinary problems/infractions Peers who use substances Being drunk in school Skipping classes Older friends Enrollment and attendance in alternative school programs supporting students at risk for school failure Intense mood changes, irritability, and anger (more than normal adolescent moodiness)

NOTE: Adapted from "Adolescent heroin abuse: Implications for the consulting professional school counselor," by G. W. Lambie and K. M. Davis, 2007, *The Journal of Professional Counseling: Practice, Theory, and Research,* 35(1), 1–17.

Additionally, professional school counselors may also use brief, adapted alcohol abuse screening approaches. An example of an effective screening procedure is CAGE (Carballo et al., 2006; Hester & Miller, 2003; Mayfield, McLeod, & Hall, 1974) where the counselors inquire of the student: Have you ever felt you needed to _Cut down_ your substance use? Have people such as your friends and family _Annoyed_ you by pestering you about your substance use? Have you ever felt _Guilty_ about your substance use? Have you ever used your substance in the morning to feel better as an _Eye-opener_? School counselors may also seek training regarding the Substance Abuse Subtle Screening Inventory—Adolescent 2 (SASSI—A2; Miller, 2001), which is a widely used substance abuse screening instrument for adolescents. Again, the purpose of introducing the CAGE and SASSI—A2 to counselors is not to suggest that they begin diagnosing student substance abuse; but rather, to offer them additional information, so they may better support their students.

Although not specifically designed for picking up cues of potential student substance abuse, the broad-based and cost-efficient screening approach, the Developmental Pathways Screening Program (DPSP), may also be useful to school counselors (Kuo, Vander Stoep, McCauley, & Kernic, 2009). It assists educators in identifying possible mental health problems such as emotional distress in elementary and middle school students. The DPSP could be used in conjunction with the above methods (CAGE and SASSI—A2).

CHILDREN OF ALCOHOLICS

Many students are living in homes where substance abuse is present, with estimates in excess of 28 million young people under 18 being exposed to familial alcohol abuse or dependence (Grant, 2000). Typically, these students' home environments are chaotic, with a lack of hierarchical structure and organization, weak parenting, poor problem-solving and interactional processes, and inappropriate emotional support (Bijttebier, Goethals, & Ansoms, 2006). Caregivers abusing alcohol often are ineffective in meeting children's educational, psychosocial, and developmental needs and add many atypical stressors to their families (Hussong, Bauer, Huang, Chassin, Sher, & Zucker, 2008; van der Zwaluw, Scholte, Vermulst, Buitelaar, Verkes, & Engels, 2008). School counselors serving as advocates and agents for systemic change (American School Counselor Association [ASCA], 2005) may support early identification and intervention for students with familial substance abuse that is "essential for breaking the systemic homeostasis of this dysfunctionality, which often leads students to fail to achieve their potential and to develop feelings of guilt, shame, and worthlessness" (Lambie & Sias, 2005, p. 272). Additionally, parental/caregiver substance abuse may be deemed as a form of child abuse and may require a school counselor to file a report with Child Protective Services in some states (Crosson-Tower, 2007).

Potential Consequences

Parental/caregiver alcohol abuse and dependence is a family illness, impacting all family members. When one family member is abusing a substance(s), all the other family members adapt to this familial dysfunction, even if it contributes to their un-healthy development (Lambie & Rokutani, 2002; van der Zwaluw et al., 2008). Research has identified multiple potential long-term behavioral, social, and psychological consequences of parental/caregiver alcohol abuse, including a four times greater propensity to develop alcohol abuse or dependence (Brooke et al., 2003); increased rates of depression, anxiety, and conduct disorders; poor and inflexible coping skills; lower levels of global self-worth (Bijttebeier et al., 2006); and increased school attrition and truancy and reduced academic achievement and standardized test scores (Kinney, 2008; Lambie & Sias, 2005). Unfortunately, only a limited number of these students receive any type of professional counseling service (Kataoka, Zhang, & Wells, 2002).

Wegscheider-Cruse (1985) identified family roles of children of alcoholics that develop as these students attempt to cope with their dysfunctional family environments (Hussong et al., 2008; Veronie & Fruehstorfer, 2001). The family roles presented in Table 5.2 are generalizations based on a person's coping mechanisms and are not intended to be used as diagnostic labels. Further, they have not been empirically validated and therefore must be used tentatively to understand the dynamics of the family constellation. Nevertheless, these family roles may offer a useful framework for counselors to understand families with alcohol abuse and dependence.

Warning Signs

Identification and thus early intervention to support children of alcoholics may be difficult because students are not likely to disclose their family secret of substance abuse. However, several behavioral signs as presented in Table 5.3 may serve well in assisting counselors in their possible identification in order to help students. However, students exhibiting behavioral cues do not indicate diagnostic pathology; rather, counselors should obtain additional information from students as they facilitate a safe and trusting environment.

RECOMMENDATIONS FOR SCHOOL
COUNSELING PRACTICE

The role of the professional school counselor is to support the academic, career, and social/personal needs of all students (ASCA, 2005). Students who abuse substances and who are children of alcoholics often need greater academic and personal-social support. Within a comprehensive school counseling program, prevention services (e.g., the large group guidance curriculum) are provided to all students with the intent of reducing potential problematic behaviors (ASCA, 2004, 2005). More specifically, NSDUH (2009b) noted that "substance use prevention programs are designed to lessen the influence of risk factors and increase the influence of protective factors" (p. 127). SAMHSA's Center for Substance Abuse Prevention (http://prevention.samhsa.gov/) provides resources and curricula for school counselors in coordinating and facilitating their substance abuse prevention services.

TABLE 5.2   Children of Alcoholics—Family Roles

Family Role	Generalized Descriptions
Chief Enabler	The chief enabler attempts to control, rationalize, minimize, and take responsibility for the family's substance abuse-related problems. Frequently, the alcohol abuser's partner.
Family Hero	Family heroes work hard to make the family appear healthy and functional. They generally are the firstborn, achievement oriented, responsible, perfectionist, parentified, and model students. Frequently, school personnel find these students to be delightful and they are natural leaders at school. Often, these students are "people pleasers" and seek the approval of others.
Family Scapegoat	Scapegoats are the opposite of the heroes, as they work to divert attention away from the parental alcohol abuse by acting out. They are often blamed for any problems and tend to be labeled the "identified client" (IC) in counseling, acting as the symptom-bearer for the family's dysfunction. These students are often labeled as rebels and troublemakers who are angry and act out at school.
Lost Child	The lost child adapts to the system's chaos by identifying with the other family members' pain, wanting to reduce it and possibly take it from them. They tend to deny their feelings and needs, internalizing their pain, which can put them at high risk for self-injurious behavior and/or suicide. Additionally, these students may have deficits in social skills because they have learned to adapt by removing themselves from situations. They are frequently seen as loners who are shy and sensitive.
Family Mascot	The family mascot's principal function is to redirect attention away from the family's alcohol abuse and pain through humor, charm, foolishness, and self-deprecation. At school these students often are the center of attention (i.e., a class clown), while in their family they try to alleviate others' pain by making them laugh. Mascots are often compassionate, possessing strong aptitudes and may be the leaders in a school's drama and music departments.

NOTE: Adapted from "Children of alcoholics: Implications for professional school counselors," by G. W. Lambie and S. M. Sias, 2005, *Professional School Counseling, 8,* 266–273.

Schools provide a logical place to identify and assist students abusing substances and children of alcoholics, since these young people spend more time at school than anywhere else. Further, "early identification and intervention hold promise for preventing future substance abuse and reducing potentially long-lasting emotional, social, behavioral, and physical problems" (Lambie & Sias, 2005, p. 270). These students require two levels of interventional support; one at the student-client level (the individual) and the other at the systemic familial level (family-based). In addition to traditional and effective school counseling response services (e.g., individual and group counseling, the large group guidance curriculum, and consultation services), there are two promising intervention strategies for counselors to use when supporting these students within a comprehensive, developmental school counseling framework: the Brief Family Systems approach (Santisteban, Suarez-Morales, Robbins,

T A B L E 5.3   Potential School-based Indicators of Children of Alcoholics

Observable Behavior Cue	Description
Absenteeism	The student's attendance may be erratic. Students may be frequently absent so they can stay home to take care of an alcohol abusing parent or caregiver.
Tardiness	These students may often be late to school because they have to take care of their siblings and the rest of the family. For example, they may have to prepare breakfast and get their siblings off to school before they can leave for school themselves.
Unkempt Appearance	The student may come to school looking disheveled and unkempt, or just inappropriately dressed, which may suggest neglect or abuse at home. Mondays are often considered "sloppy days."
Inconsistent Performance	The student's school performance often varies from day to day, and even throughout the day. There is little consistency in these young people's lives, and this may be evident in their inconsistent behavior and mood. These students may perform better in their morning classes, but as the school day comes to an end, their functioning may deteriorate as they become distressed about returning to the home.
Poor Impulse Control	Some students may be prone to emotional outbursts, temper tantrums or other disruptive behavior, while others may demand extra attention by acting out or becoming the class clown.
Caregiver Concerns	Caregivers/parents may be difficult to reach and may fail to keep meetings and conference appointments, and may appear uninterested in their child's school performance. Additionally, the caregiver or parent may attend meetings and school functions while under the influence of alcohol.
Physical Symptoms	These students may have psychosomatic responses; that is, their emotional pain may be manifested in physical symptoms. Therefore, these students may persistently complain about stomachaches, headaches, and other physical ailments without explainable causes.
Sad Affect	These students are experiencing emotional pain. They may internalize this pain and appear to school personnel as being sad, depressed, and withdrawn.
Disciplinary Problems	Some students may internalize their pain, while others externalize. The externalizers tend to appear angry and are often involved in school disciplinary procedures for acting out, fighting, and being aggressive.
Peer Cues	The student's peers may offer hints that there is a problem. They may come to the school counselor or teacher and express concern about their friend and say that he or she is sad. Other students may tease the student for his or her caregiver's alcohol abuse.

NOTE: Adapted from "Children of alcoholics: Implications for professional school counselors," by G. W. Lambie and S. M. Sias, 2005, *Professional School Counseling, 8,* 266–273.

Szapocznik, 2006; Szapocznik, Hervis, & Schwartz, 2003) and Motivational Counseling (Miller & Rollnick, 2002; Miller, Zweben, DiClemente, & Rychtarik, 1995). Both are described in greater detail in the following section.

Brief Family Systems Approach

Crespi and Rueckert (2006) noted that both substance abusers and children of alcoholics can benefit from family systems therapeutic interventions, even when the parent/caregiver who is a substance abuser is unwilling to seek treatment. Further, the research has found that family-based intervention approaches are effective in treating school-age substance abusers (Hogue, Liddle, & Dauber, 2004). However, many school counselors have not been trained in either substance abuse or family systems therapeutic interventions (Council for Accreditation of Counseling and Related Educational Programs, 2009; Lambie & Rotutani, 2002). Therefore, the following section introduces family systems-level intervention strategies that a counselor may implement to support these students.

The Brief Family Systems Approach (BFSA) is grounded on four theoretical constructs: (a) *circularity* is where family members are interdependent and have a reciprocal relationship causing a family member to exhibit problem behavior (e.g., student abusing substances as the symptom-bearer), which indicates the dysfunctionality of the entire family system; (b) *complementarity* is the premise that "problems" are manifested in dysfunctional interactional patterns, where all family members contribute to the problem and can "fix" the problem; (c) *homeostasis* is where all systems work to maintain equilibrium, functional or dysfunctional, and thus families tend to be "stuck" in fixed interactional patterns making change difficult; and (d) *facilitating systemic change* is when a student's substance abuse problem is directly related to dysfunctional familial interactional patterns and the counselor's primary focus is on changing the interactional processes that are maintaining the maladaptive behavior (Goldenberg & Goldenberg, 2007; Szapocznik, et al., 2003). Consequently, the two primary goals of this intervention are to work to eliminate the student's problematic behavior (symptom reduction) and to facilitate second order systemic change; thus, altering the family's structure and interactional patterns associated with the student's substance abuse. The following are the strategies a counselor may implement to intervene in a student's substance abuse when using this intervention.

Joining Students' problematic behaviors tend to engender labeling them as the "problem," when from a family systems perspective, they are simply manifesting symptomology that is grounded in familial dysfunctionality. For this reason, to support both students and the change process, modification of these dysfunctional familial interactional processes is necessary. Therefore, counselors need to engage the student's family in the change process. *Joining* is when counselors work to enter the family's frame of reference as they support the development of a safe and trusting therapeutic relationship with the family. As Minuchin and Fishman (1981) noted: "Joining is the glue that holds the therapeutic system together" (p. 32). Counselors join the family from a one-down position, asking the family to help them understand the family, as they communicate respect, understanding, and an attitude that expresses that they are working for them and with them.

Focus on Process Versus Content   A primary distinction of BFSA from traditional non-systemic counseling interventions is its focus on interactional processes, and not on content or "what" the student-client and family say. Instead, this intervention focuses on the established interactional processes between family members, including how they talk to one-another, the degree of emotional expression and nurturance, and familial organization. The counselor first identifies the family's repetitive interactional patterns through observing family level behavioral interactions. Once these entrenched interaction processes are identified, the counselor works to change them through various family intervention strategies, such as unbalancing, enactments, restructuring, boundary-making, and reframing. For additional clarification regarding specific family systems counseling techniques, a review of Minuchin and Fishman (1981) and Goldenberg and Goldenberg (2007) is suggested.

Familial Education   An underlying belief within this framework is that students and families are "doing the best they can" and are simply "stuck" employing interactional processes that are not functional. Therefore, the counselor must work to change the family's interactional processes to facilitate the improved functionality of all family members. This may involve educating family members about what supports increased family functionality (e.g., adaptivity, flexibility, established hierarchical order and boundaries). For many families with substance abuse issues, this may involve educating the familial hierarchy (parents or adult caregivers) about appropriate parental roles. The research has consistently indicated that poor parental/caregiver nurturance and support, a conflict-based parent/caregiver–child relationship and communication, and inappropriate familial hierarchical structure, such as overly authoritative and rigid or inconsistent and passive, are positively correlated with student substance abuse (Juhnke & Hagedorn, 2006; Lambie & Rotutani, 2002). Therefore, parent/caregiver education may serve as both a prevention and intervention strategy to support these students.

Serve as a Systemic Liaison   The intent of introducing this intervention is not to suggest that counselors should begin offering family counseling services to all the families they serve; but rather, to offer an orientation to a family systems perspective of student substance abuse related issues. Within this framework, school counselors may effectively serve as liaisons among the systemic organizations that maintain or intervene in a student's maladaptive behavior (e.g., school, outside agencies, and the family). It is important to note that school counselors should not "blame" either the family or student for their "problem" as this tends to evoke resistance (Lambie, 2004). Rather, they should focus on facilitating future change and self-efficacy. For example, in the case study of Jeff, the counselor may ask: "Well, we know Jeff has been struggling recently, but what do you think each of us may do to support Jeff in being successful?"

Motivational Counseling

Motivational Counseling (MC) is an integration of Motivational Interviewing (Miller & Rollnick, 2002) and Motivational Enhancement Therapy (Miller et al.,

1995), and incorporates the Transtheoretical Model of Change (TMC; Prochaska, DiClemente, & Norcross, 1992), which was designed to help clients build commitment and achieve behavioral change. MC has been found to be effective with young people with substance abuse related problems (Carroll et al., 2006; Lambie, 2004; Stein et al., 2006; Stern, Meredith, Gholson, Gore, & D'Amico, 2007). Additionally, Stein and colleagues (2007) concluded that MC is "particularly useful for clients who are reluctant to change…" (p. 305). This intervention type draws on strategies from client-centered counseling, cognitive therapy, systems theory, and the social psychology of persuasion (Miller & Rollnick, 2002). Some features of MC include motivation to change that is elicited from the student and brief in duration; direct persuasion is avoided; the style is generally quiet and eliciting; readiness to change is seen as fluctuating in relation to interpersonal interaction; it emphasizes the student's self-determination and power of choice; and the counseling relationship is more like a partnership or companionship than expert/recipient roles (Ingersoll, Wagner, & Gharib, 2006; Lambie, 2004).

Transtheoretical Model of Change   TMC is grounded on research and focuses on how people change. Prochaska and colleagues (1992) proposed that people who change their behaviors—whether on their own or with the help of a counselor—tend to go through five stages of change, frequently using different processes or methods at various stages. These five stages (as cited in Lambie, 2004) are:

1. *Precontemplation.* Students don't consider their behavior to be a problem and/or are not currently considering changing their behavior.
2. *Contemplation.* Students are beginning to consider that their behavior may be a problem and are seriously thinking of, or contemplating, changing their behavior.
3. *Preparation.* Students have made a commitment to change a behavior they consider problematic and are intending to make the change soon, and they may already have a specific plan in mind.
4. *Action.* Students are currently in the process of modifying their behavior or environment to reduce or eliminate the problem identified. They are considered to be in the action stage for up to six months following the initial behavior change (assuming that they maintain the change during the period).
5. *Maintenance.* Students work to prevent a return to the problem behavior and to stabilize the new behaviors and/or environment that supports their new way of living.

This intervention regards change as difficult, in which linear progression is possible, but is relatively rare. Thus, it offers a spiral pattern of the stages of change where people can progress from contemplation to preparation to action, but most people will lapse to an earlier stage at some point. This can guide the counselor to more successful outcomes by matching counseling processes to the student's individual level of readiness to change. This model advocates that counselors adapt their counseling to the stage where the student actually is in the change process.

At the lower stages of change (precontemplation and contemplation), the counselor works to reduce possible resistance by using nondirective counseling techniques such as asking open-ended questions, listening reflectively, affirming, and summarizing. As the student moves to the higher stages of change (preparation, action, and maintenance), the counselor becomes more directive and behavioral by assisting the student in developing and implementing a plan for behavioral change (Ingersoll et al., 2006; Miller & Rollnick, 2002). When working with a student in precontemplation or contemplation stage, the counselor is like a caring, empathic caregiver/parent. As the student moves to the subsequent stages, the counselor becomes a supportive coach supplying more behavioral direction.

MC Therapeutic Strategies   This approach is designed to help people work through their ambivalence about change, primarily through the use of active listening and gentle feedback techniques. The goal is to prepare people for change, and the counselor's task is to create conditions that enhance the student's motivation for and commitment to change, not necessarily to coerce him or her into changing right away (Miller et al., 1995). This strategy seeks to support an intrinsic motivation for change, which leads the student to initiate, persist in, and comply with behavior change efforts.

Miller and Rollnick (2002) listed six basic motivational tenets underlying the MC approach. These motivational principles include:

1. *Expression of empathy and respect.* The counselor communicates respect for students and listens rather than tells.

2. *Assisting students in perceiving discrepancy.* The counselor uses motivational psychology principles to help students perceive a discrepancy between where they are and where they want to be.

3. *Avoiding argumentation.* When a counselor directly confronts and argues with a student-client, it evokes resistance, defined as a student's reactions to a perceived threatening interpersonal interaction, which is known as psychological reactance (Brehm & Brehm, 1981)

4. *Rolling with resistance.* The counselor does not meet resistance head on, but rather "rolls with" the momentum, with a goal of shifting student perceptions in the process.

5. *Ambivalence is viewed as normal and openly discussed.* The counselor elicits solutions from the student in order to reduce ambivalence to change.

6. *Support of the student's sense of self-efficacy.* The counselor works to enhance the student's perceived ability to achieve his or her own goals. People only move towards change when they believe that there is a chance of success.

MC also offers other strategies that may be effective for school counselors working with students; however, reviewing each of these strategies is beyond the scope of this chapter. Readers who are interested might consult these excellent resources: Brook and McHenry (2009), Ingersoll et al. (2006), Lambie (2004), Miller et al. (1995), Miller and Rollnick (2002).

SUMMARY

Students abusing substances and children of alcoholics are in all schools and require school-based prevention and intervention strategies to support their holistic development. This chapter presented professional school counselors an orientation to common substance abuse related issues students frequently struggle with and listed therapeutic intervention approaches that have been found effective for supporting these students. However, as the National Institute on Drug Abuse (1999) noted, "no single treatment is appropriate for all individuals … treatment needs to be readily available … effective treatment attends to multiple needs of the individual, not just his or her drug use" (p. 3).

Prevention of substance abuse-related problems is preferred to remediation and treatment. ASCA (2005) advocates comprehensive, developmental school counseling programs that are proactive and preventive in nature, rather than reactive. Watkins, Ellickson, Vaiana, and Hiromoto (2006) concluded that substance abuse prevention "can be effective, but only if counselors convey credible and age-appropriate information" (p. 136). For additional information regarding substance abuse prevention programs, readers should consult Table 5.4 as well as the SAMHSA's Center for Substance Abuse Prevention (www.prevention.samhsa.gov/about/) and the Substance Abuse and Mental Health Services Administration (www.samhsa.gov).

Professional school counselors are certified/licensed educational professionals with specialized training who serve as advocates and agents for systemic change to support all students' achievements and success (ASCA, 2005). To support all

T A B L E 5.4   Additional Resources

Al-Anon	www.al-anon.org
Alateen	www.alateen.org
Alcoholics Anonymous	www.alcoholics-anonymous.org
Center for Substance Abuse Prevention	www.prevention.samhsa.gov/about/
Drug Resistance Abuse Education	www.dare.com
Motivational Interviewing	www.motivationalinterviewing.org
The National Association for Children of Alcoholics	www.nacoa.org
The National Student Assistance Association	www.nasap.org
The National Council on Alcoholism and Drug Dependence	www.ncadd.org
The National Institute on Alcohol Abuse and Alcoholism	www.niaaa.nih.gov
The National Institute on Drug Abuse	www.nida.nih.gov
Substance Abuse and Mental Health Services Administration	www.samhsa.gov
U.S. Department of Health and Human Services and SAMHSA's National Clearinghouse for Alcohol & Drug Information	www.ncadi.samhsa.gov

students, school counselors must appreciate and understand the potential, significantly negative influence familial and student substance abuse has on young people. If counselors did not receive any training relating to substance abuse in their preparation program, they have an ethical obligation to seek additional professional development to increase their professional competencies. The intent of this chapter is to serve as an initiation for school counselors in their development to support students impacted by substance abuse-related issues.

REFERENCES

American Psychiatric Association. (2000). *Diagnostic and statistical manual of mental disorders* (4th ed., text rev.). Washington DC: Author.

American School Counselor Association. (2004). *Position statement: The professional school counselor and the prevention and intervention of behaviors that practice students at risk.* Alexandria, VA: Author.

American School Counselor Association. (2005). *The ASCA national model: A framework for school counseling programs* (2nd ed.). Alexandria, VA: Author.

Bijttebier, P., Goethals, E., & Ansoms, S. (2006). Parental drinking as a risk factor for children's maladjustment: The mediating role of family environment. *Psychology of Addictive Behavior, 20,* 126–130.

Brehm, S. S., & Brehm, J. W. (1981). *Psychological reactance: A theory of freedom and control.* New York: Academic Press.

Brook, D. W., Brook, J. S., Rubenstone, E., Zhang, C., Singer, M., & Duke, M. R. (2003). Alcohol use in adolescents whose fathers abuse drugs. *Journal of Addictive Disease, 2*(1), 11–43.

Brook, F., & McHenry, B. (2009). *A contemporary approach to substance abuse and addiction counseling: A counselor's guide to application and understanding.* Alexandria, VA: American Counseling Association.

Brook, J. S., Saar, N. S., Zhang, C., & Brook, D. W. (2009). Psychosocial antecedent and adverse health consequences related to substance use. *American Journal of Public Health, 99,* 563–568.

Carballo, J. J., Oquendo, M. A., Giner, L., Garcia-Parajua, P., Iglesias, J. J., Goldber, H., et al. (2006). Prevalence of alcohol misuse among adolescents and young adults evaluated in primary care settings. *International Journal of Adolescent Medicine and Health, 18*(1), 197–2002.

Carroll, K. M., Ball, S. A., Nich, C., Martino, S., Frankforter, T. L., Farentinos, C., et al. (2006). Motivational interviewing to improve treatment engagement and outcome in individuals seeking treatment for substance abuse: A multisite effectiveness study. *Drug and Alcohol Dependence, 81,* 301–312.

Council for Accreditation of Counseling and Related Educational Programs. (2009). *CACREP accreditation standards and procedures manual.* Alexandria, VA: Author.

Crespi, T. D., & Rueckert, Q. H. (2006). Family therapy and children of alcoholics: Implications for continuing education and certification in substance abuse practice. *Journal of Child & Adolescent Substance Abuse, 15*(3), 33–44.

Crosson-Tower, C. (2007). *Understanding child abuse and neglect* (7th ed.). Boston: Allyn and Bacon.

Deas, D., Roberts, J. S., & Grindlinger, D. (2005). The utility of DSM–IV criteria in diagnosing substance abuse/dependence in adolescents. *Journal of Substance Use, 10*(1), 10–21.

Eaton, D. K., Brener, N., & Kann, L. K. (2007). Associations of health risk behaviors with school absenteeism. Does having permission for the absence make a difference? *Journal of School Health, 78,* 223–229.

Goldenberg, H., & Goldenberg, I. (2007). *Family therapy: An overview* (7th ed.). Belmont, CA: Thomas Brook/Cole.

Grant, G. F. (2000). Estimates of US children exposed to alcohol abuse and dependence in the family. *American Journal of Public Health, 90*(1), 112–116.

Hester, R. K., & Miller, W. R. (2003). *Handbook of alcoholism treatment approaches: Effective alternatives* (3rd ed.). Boston: Pearson Education.

Hogue, A., Liddle, H. A., & Dauber, S. (2004). Linking session focus to treatment outcome in evidence-based treatments for adolescent substance abuse. *Psychotherapy: Theory, Practice, and Training, 41*(2), 83–96.

Hussong, A. M., Bauer, D. J., Huang, W., Chassin, L., Sher, K. J., & Zucker, R. A. (2008). Characterizing the life stressors of children of alcoholic parents. *Journal of Family Psychology, 22,* 819–832.

Ingersoll, K. S., Wagner, C. C., & Gharib, S. (2006). *Motivational groups for community substance abuse programs* (3rd ed.). Richmond, VA: Mid-Atlantic Addiction Technology Transfer Center.

Johnston, L. D., O'Malley, P. M., Bachman, J. G., & Schulenberg, J. E. (2006). *Monitoring the future national results on adolescent drug use: Overview of key findings, 2005* (NIH Publication No. 06–5882). Bethesda, MD: National Institute on Drug Abuse.

Juhnke, G., & Hagedorn, W. B. (2006). *Counseling addicted families: An integrative assessment and treatment model.* New York: Routledge Taylor & Francis Group.

Kataoka, S. H., Zhang, L., & Wells, K. B. (2002). Unmet need for mental health care among U.S. children: Variation by ethnicity and insurance status. *American Journal of Psychiatry, 159,* 1548–1555.

Kuo, E., Vander Stoep, A., McCauley, E., & Kernic, M. A. (2009). Cost-effectiveness of a school-based emotional health screening program. *Journal of School Health, 79,* 277–285.

Kinney, J. (2008). *Loosening the grip: A handbook of alcohol information* (9th ed.). Columbus, OH: McGraw-Hill.

Lambie, G. W. (2004). Motivational Enhancement Therapy: A tool for professional school counselors working with adolescents. *Professional School Counseling, 7,* 268–276.

Lambie, G. W., & Davis, K. M. (2007). Adolescent heroin abuse: Implications for the consulting professional school counselor. *The Journal of Professional Counseling: Practice, Theory, and Research, 35*(1), 1–17.

Lambie, G., & Rokutani, L. (2002). A systems approach to substance abuse identification and intervention for school counselors. *Professional School Counseling, 5*(5), 353–359.

Lambie, G. W., & Sias, S. M. (2005). Children of alcoholics: Implications for professional school counseling. *Professional School Counseling, 8,* 266–273.

Lambie, G. W., & Smith, T. W. (2004). Adolescent substance abuse: A practical resource for teachers. *The South Carolina Middle School Journal, 7*(1), 30–32.

Mayfield, D., McLeod, G., & Hall, P. (1974). The CAGE questionnaire: Validation of a new alcoholism screening instrument. *American Journal of Psychiatry, 131,* 1121–1123.

Miller, F. G. (2001). *The SASSI–A2 manual.* Spring, IN: SASSI Institute.

Miller, W. R., & Rollnick, S. (2002). *Motivational interviewing: Preparing people to change addictive behavior* (2nd ed.). New York: Guilford.

Miller, W. R., Zweben, A., DiClemente, C. C. & Rychtarik, R. G. (1995). *Motivational Enhancement Therapy manual: A clinical research guide for therapists treating individuals with alcohol abuse and dependence* (Volume 2, Project MATCH Monograph Series). Rockville, MD: National Institute of Alcohol Abuse and Alcoholism.

Minuchin, S., & Fishman, H. C. (1981). *Family therapy techniques.* Boston: Harvard University Press. National Institute on Drug Abuse. (1999). *Principles of drug addiction treatment: A research-based guide.* Rockville, MD: Author.

National Survey on Drug Use and Health. (2006). *The NSDUH report: Academic performance and substance use among students ages 12 to 17: 2002, 2003, and 2004.* Retrieved November 18, 2006, from http://www.oas.samhsa.gov/2k6/academics/academics.pdf

National Survey on Drug Use and Health. (2008). *The NSDUH report: Trends in substance use, dependence or abuse, and treatment among adolescents: 2002 to 2007.* Retrieved June 4, 2009, from http://oas.samhsa.gov/2k8/youthTrends/youthTrends.pdf

National Survey on Drug Use and Health. (2009a). *The NSDUH report: Children living with substance-dependent or substance-abusing parents: 2002 to 2007.* Retrieved June 4, 2009, from http://oas.samhsa.gov/2k9/SAparents/SAparents.pdf

National Survey on Drug Use and Health. (2009b). *The NSDUH report: Exposure to substance use prevention messages and substance use among adolescents: 2002 to 2007.* Retrieved June 4, 2009, http://oas.samhsa.gov/2k9/prevention/prevention.pdf

Palmer, R. H. C., Young, S. E., et al. (2009). Developmental epidemiology of drug use and abuse in adolescence and young adulthood: Evidence of generalized risk. *Drug & Alcohol Dependence, 102,* 78–87.

Prochaska, J. O., DiClemente, C. C., & Norcross, J. C. (1992). In search of how people change: Applications to addictive behavior. *American Psychologist, 47,* 1102–1114.

Santisteban, D. A., Suarez-Morales, L., Robbins, M. S., & Szapocznik, J. (2006). Brief strategic family therapy: Lessons learned in efficacy research and challenges to blending research and practice. *Family Process, 45,* 259–271.

Stein, L. A. R., Colby, S. M., Barnett, N. P., Monti, P. M., Golembeske, C., Lebveau-Craven, R., Miranda, R. (2006). Enhancing substance abuse treatment engagement in incarcerated adolescents. *Psychological Services, 3*(1), 25–34.

Stern, S. A., Meredith, L. S., Gholson, J., Gore, P., & D'Amico, E. J. (2007). Project CHAT: A brief motivational substance abuse intervention for teens in primary care. *Journal of Substance Abuse Treatment, 32,* 153–165.

Substance Abuse and Mental Health Services Administration. (2008). *Results from the 2007 National Survey on Drug Use and Health: National Findings* (Office of Applied Studies, NSDUH Series H–34, DHHS Publication No. SMA 08–4343). Rockville, MD.

Szapocznik, J., Hervis, O., & Schwartz, S. (2003). *Therapy manual for drug addiction: Brief Strategic Family Therapy for adolescent drug abuse.* Bethesda, MD: National Institute of Drug Abuse.

van der Zwaluw, C. S., Scholte, R.H. J., Vermulst, A.A., Buitelaar, J. K., Verkes, R. J., & Engels, R. C. (2008). Parental problem drinking, parenting, and adolescent alcohol use. *Journal of Behavioral Medicine, 31,* 189–200.

Veronie, L., & Fruehstorfer, D. B. (2001). Gender, birth order, and family role identification among adult children of alcoholics. *Current Psychology: Developmental, Learning, Personality, Social, 20*(1), 53–67.

Watkins, K. E., Ellickson, P. L., Vaiana, M. E., & Hiromoto, S. (2006). An update on adolescent drug use: What school counselors need to know? *Professional School Counseling, 10,* 131–138.

Wegscheider-Cruse, S. (1985). *Choice-making.* Pompano Beach, FL: Health Communications.

Chapter 6

Child Sexual Abuse

CAROLYN STONE

University of North Florida

S chool counselors, as consultants, are well situated to provide an awareness to teachers and other educators of developmental sexual behavior and the symptoms of sexual abuse (Brown, Brack, & Mullis, 2008). Over the course of their career, school counselors will see dozens of students who appear to lead normal, happy lives when behind closed doors their lives may be a secret nightmare. Hopefully, school counselors are able to promote healthy sexual development for students through their role as consultant, leader, advocate, counselor, and coordinator. Knowledge of intervention and prevention techniques allow the professional school counselor to provide leadership in helping more children develop into happy healthy adults.

This chapter provides prevention and intervention strategies through the analysis of case studies and will help the school counseling professional recognize the signs and symptoms of child sexual abuse or neglect and understand the legal

---

Sarah: A School-Based Case Study

Sarah's kindergarten teacher reports the elementary school counselor that Sarah is exhibiting some disturbing sexual behaviors. She talks about adult sexual activities, she touches other students in inappropriate ways, talks about her peers' body parts, and she has been masturbating in class. Both the teacher and counselor are concerned because they are not sure if this is a case of Sarah being a victim of sexual abuse or perhaps a developmental stage, even though it is inappropriate behavior for a school setting.

and ethical dimensions of this often hidden problem. The cases involve sexual issues that school counselors frequently find themselves being asked to address in order to ensure students a safe and respectful childhood.

This is a situation in which the professional school counselor, as consultant, will struggle to find the right interventions; but without question, an intervention is needed. Let's explore the challenging scenario. Obviously this case asks for the school counselor's best judgment of whether child abuse reporting needs to be considered. Sample questions to ponder when working with Sarah are: Is this developmentally the sexual behavior of a kindergartener? Is this a matter for Child Protective Services (CPS), requiring a phone call? Is this a consultation scenario where the counselor should assist the teacher with Sarah's "normal" behaviors, as they are inappropriate for the classroom? Should a referral be made to an outside agency for extreme behaviors that require intensive interventions (Wilder, 1991)?

DEFINING DEVELOPMENTALLY NORMAL SEXUAL BEHAVIOR IN CHILDREN

Is Sarah's behavior in the case study developmentally normal sexual behavior? Research about children's developmental sexual behavior is limited, but what is known is that children's normal sexual behavior includes curiosity, interest, and experimentation, and it progresses over time (Bancroft, 2003; Gil & Johnson, 1993; James & Burch, 1999). Childhood sexuality coincides with physical, emotional, psychological, cognitive, and moral development (Gil & Johnson; James & Burch). For specific examples, the American Academy of Pediatrics (AAP, n.d.) listed "normal" to "rarely normal" sexual behaviors demonstrated by children ages 2 through 6 years. In the case of Sarah, it is common that a child her age would be curious about private parts and may sporadically engage in mild masturbation. Beginning in preschool, children may touch the genitals of playmates and/or become involved in undressing games. They are interested in showing and viewing their private parts. Kindergarteners are generally aware of physical differences and are curious about the human body. It is not uncommon to hear them use slang words for body parts and bathroom-related behaviors. This age group may also act repulsed by sexual behaviors they see on television, while at the same time, remain curious about them (AAP; Bancroft; Gil & Johnson; James & Burch).

Evaluating Children's Sexual Behaviors

Abused children's sexual behavior can extend beyond normal developmental sexual curiosity (Brown et al. 2008; James & Burch, 1999). The research of Einbender and Friedrich (1989) reported on the sexual preoccupation of sexually abused girls (as compared to a group of non-abused girls who were congruous in age, family income, and race). Thus, intense preoccupation with sex is considered to be a key indicator of sexual abuse in children (Chromy, 2007; Hall, Mathews, & Pearce, 1998). When interviewed, parents of sexually abused children report that their children think and talk too much about sex (Kelly, 1993). Abused children's sexual behavior involves power and aggression (Hall et al.; Gil & Johnson, 1993). Children may masturbate to the point of soreness or rub or poke themselves with play items and may expose themselves more frequently (White & Allers, 1994; Gil & Johnson). The play theme of abused children may be highly unusual with compulsive, excited sexual content (Brown et al.; Curry & Arnaud, 1995). Children also express sexual abuse through artwork and drawings (Sadowski & Loesch, 1993; Tillman, 2004).

To determine if Sarah is a victim of child sexual abuse or merely exhibiting curious or developmentally appropriate behavior, it is important to look for more than one symptom. It is a good idea to err on the side of caution: If in doubt, report the case to Child Protective Services. Readers should note that a thorough list of child sexual abuse indicators is provided on several reputable Web sites (e.g., American Academy of Child and Adolescent Psychiatry, 2008; Child Welfare Information Gateway, 2008a).

If Sarah is "merely" exhibiting developmentally appropriate sexual behavior, school counselors can offer support to the teachers and other adults in the child's life. The first effort should be to inform all the adults about what is considered normal childhood sexual development. The following are suggestions from James and Burch (1999) as to how to respond to normal childhood sexual development.

- Avoid severely reprimanding or punishing children's sexual behavior.
- Promote other activities. For example, a teacher can interrupt sexual behavior by asking a child to run errands. Or, if a child is masturbating at naptime because of boredom, the teacher may give the child a quiet game or puzzle.
- Be matter-of-fact and answer questions about sexual matters in an assuring, firm manner without shaming children. For instance, an adult might confirm that masturbation is a normal, yet private, activity.
- Put limits on the touching of others' genitals.
- Prevent children from watching adult sexual activity.
- Talk to parents and guardians about outside counseling if you think a child is exhibiting excessive behavior, such as masturbating more than usual. The behavior may be caused by fear or anxiety.
- Keep accurate, objective records of the child's behavior, contact with parents, referrals, and school interventions.
- Be alert to your own demeanor, especially if you feel nervousness, fear, disapproval, shock, or anger.
- Consult with more experienced colleagues.

Level of Incidence of Sexual Issues

According to *Child Maltreatment 2004* (see "Summary: What types of maltreatment were found?"), a report from the National Child Abuse and Neglect Data System (NCANDS; Children's Bureau, 2009b), approximately 872,000 children were found to be victims of child abuse or neglect in calendar year 2004. Of this number, roughly 60% suffered parental or caregiver neglect, 18% were physically abused, 10% were sexually abused, 7% were emotionally or psychologically maltreated, and 2% were medically neglected. Additionally, 15% of victims experienced "other" types of maltreatment such as "abandonment," "threats of harm to the child," and "congenital drug addiction" (Children's Bureau, 2009b).

It is difficult to gauge the accuracy of the number of child abuse and neglect incidents, as the data only reflect the number of cases actually reported. The *Child Maltreatment 2004* report tracking data from 1990 to 2004 indicates that while the abuse investigation rate has gradually increased (about 27%) over time, the victimization rate has somewhat declined (7.5%; Children's Bureau, 2009a). Regrettably, trend data are not altogether clear for child sexual abuse, but evidence drawn from 1992–2000 data shows a modest decline as well (Finkelhor & Jones, 2004). More recently, Child Maltreatment 2007 data reported an overall incidence rate 7.6% for childhood sexual abuse (see http://www.acf.hhs.gov/programs/cb/pubs/cm07/table3_8.htm).

SIGNS OF SEXUAL ABUSE IN CHILDREN

It is important to note that no one single sign is typically indicative of child sexual abuse. Rather, when these signs occur repeatedly and in combination, an alert professional school counselor may consider child abuse as a possible cause. The following should be considered as signs of possible child sexual abuse. The child:

- has difficulty walking or sitting.
- suddenly refuses to change for gym or to participate in physical activities.
- reports nightmares or bed-wetting.
- experiences a sudden change in appetite.
- demonstrates bizarre, sophisticated, or unusual sexual knowledge or behavior.
- becomes pregnant or contracts a venereal disease, particularly if under age 14.
- runs away.
- reports sexual abuse by a parent or another adult caregiver.

Consider the possibility of sexual abuse when the parent or other adult caregiver:

- is unduly protective of the child or severely limits the child's contact with other children, especially of the opposite sex.
- is secretive and isolated.

- is jealous or controlling of family members. (Child Welfare Information Gateway, 2007)

Often there are no obvious physical signs of sexual abuse. Some signs can only be detected by a physician during a physical exam. Sexually abused children may develop the following:

- unusual interest in or avoidance of all things of a sexual nature
- sleep problems or nightmares
- depression or withdrawal from friends or family
- seductiveness
- statements that their bodies are dirty or damaged, or fear that there is something wrong with them in the genital area
- refusal to go to school
- delinquency/conduct problems
- secretiveness
- aspects of sexual molestation in drawings, games, fantasies
- unusual aggressiveness, or
- suicidal behavior. (American Academy of Child and Adolescent Psychiatry, 2008)

Student Disclosure

When a student's sexual abuse is made known it is most likely because the child disclosed their sexual victimization (DeVoe & Faller, 1999). Unfortunately, studies of adults who were sexually abused during childhood indicate that the majority never told anyone of their victimization (Fieldman & Crespi, 2002; London, Bruck, Ceci, & Shuman, 2005). When a child reveals abuse to an educator, it should trigger a call to protective services.

The disclosure can be an evolving process in which the student reveals, then recants or makes hints, and then denies (Berliner & Conte, 1995; London et al.). Sorenson and Snow (1991) analyzed children's sexual abuse disclosures and found that only 11% of the children disclosed the sexual abuse they had endured, without denial, in the initial investigative interview. Of the children in the study, 22% recanted their sexual abuse reports at the initial interview, and 92% subsequently reaffirmed their allegations. Following this study, a review of sexual abuse reporting literature showed that "approximately 60%–70% of adults [who were sexually abused as children] do not recall ever disclosing their abuse as children, and only a small minority of participants (10%–18%) recalled that their cases were reported to the authorities" (London et al., 2005, p. 203).

Other important information about student disclosure:

- Over 30% of victims never disclose their experience to anyone (Darkness to Light, 2008).

- Young victims may not recognize their victimization as sexual abuse and younger children may be less likely to disclose than older children (London et al., 2005).

- Almost 80% initially deny abuse or are tentative in disclosing. Of those who do disclose, approximately 75% disclose accidentally. Additionally, of those who do disclose, more than 20% eventually recant even though the abuse occurred (Darkness to Light). But by at least the second investigative interview, only a small minority of children recant their abuse reports (London et al.).

- Once children have made an abuse disclosure, they are likely to maintain their allegations during formal assessments (London et al.).

- Fabricated sexual abuse reports constitute only 1% to 4% of all reported cases. Of these, 75% are false reports by adults and 25% are by children. Children only fabricate .5% of the time (Darkness to Light).

Interviewing Potential Victims of Child Sexual Abuse

Often, possible child sexual abuse will come to the counselor's attention through a teacher referral, and there are appropriate methods to use and numerous resources to consult as he or she conducts the interview with the student (e.g., Pipe & Salmon, 2009). When meeting children who may have been sexually abused, school counselors will benefit from using nonverbal interview props (e.g., dolls, drawings, body diagrams, etc.) and techniques (Pipe & Salmon, 2009) as well as verbal methods. Short and open style rapport-building techniques and supportive dialogue are associated with richer information gained from children's responses (Hershkowitz, 2009). Examples of appropriate questions would be: "Can you tell me about a time when something happened to you that made you feel uncomfortable?" (England & Thompson, 1988, p. 372), or simply "What has happened to you?" (Zuckerman, 1993, p. 27). Avoid using long and complex sentences, multiple questions at one time, and vague references to persons and circumstances (Korkman, Santtila, Drzewiecki, & Sandnabba, 2007). Obviously, watch the child for both verbal and nonverbal responses. The child's body language during the interview can reveal more than words in some cases. School counselors' skills at attending will be useful.

Allow the child to unfold the story at his or her own pace without leading them down any particular path. It is vitally important to avoid asking leading questions, as defense lawyers representing the alleged abuser in court may attempt to make a case that you contaminated the testimony of the alleged abuse victim. This will hinder any potential prosecution and may lead the child down the road to telling untruths about his or her experiences. Contamination can include asking leading questions, feeding the child information, helping the child with details, asking numerous questions, or pressuring. School counselors should not make their investigation through an exhaustive interview (Stone, 2005).

According to an American School Counselor Association (2003) position statement on this topic, the purpose of an interview is to gather information for a report of suspected child abuse and to help the child, not to establish proof of abuse or to determine cause. If the school counselor has a reasonable suspicion, then this is enough to establish that a phone call to child protective services is required, and the interview stops. The school counselor may support the student with unconditional positive regard but must cease interviewing. In many states a student may only be interviewed a finite number of times, and this interview could in some states be counted as one of those limited number of interviews. Remember, the only thing a counselor is trying to determine is reasonable suspicion, not the facts of the case. Other potential legal and ethical issues at stake are discussed next.

LEGAL AND ETHICAL ISSUES IN REPORTING CHILD SEXUAL ABUSE

The Professional School Counselor and Child Abuse and Neglect Prevention position statement (ASCA, 2003) states that "It is the professional school counselor's legal, ethical and moral responsibility to report suspected cases of child abuse/neglect to the proper authorities" (p. 4).

Being mandated by law to report suspected cases of child sexual abuse means that one must be aware and alert to the potential of abuse and then evaluate its presence (Stone 2005). School counselors must be willing to identify and also acknowledge the signs of abuse and be brave enough to take action, knowing that there is tremendous support for them both in the law and in their ethical codes. School counselors can also admit that there is fear associated with reporting abuse but are reminded that their feelings of fear as an adult are magnified greatly for abused children who have no control over their situation. Children are our most vulnerable citizens, and good judgment and courage to care for them is the professional school counselor's mandate.

Child sexual abuse can be notoriously insidious and cannot always be definitively identified. It is the gray area that is worrisome. Being a mandatory reporter requires considered judgment (Brown et al. 2008). In matters of family and the sanctity of the home, due process of thought is needed. Decisions concerning child sexual abuse almost always move into areas of judgment and degrees. Some cases are simple; the evidence is irrefutable and conclusive. Sexual abuse can fall into this category.

The school counselor as a mandated reporter knows the devastating effect of child sexual abuse and wants to report it; yet, the fallout from a false report is enormous. The counselor must exercise prudence in deciding which path to take. However, caution is necessary. Weigh the consequences of reporting. Which is the bigger hurt—reporting a suspected case of child sexual abuse and finding out you were wrong, or not reporting it and finding out you were right? Err on the side of caution. Reasonable suspicion is all that is required in order to report suspected abuse (Brown et al.; Stone, 2005).

Legal Responsibilities

State statutes vary slightly in language, but the meaning is generally the same and reads similarly. Educators and counselors are mandatory child abuse reporters, which means that they:

- *have an absolute duty to report.*
- do not have to be certain; suspicion is enough to establish a duty.
- have a duty that is not discretionary; it is inextricably clear.
- have an obligation to make their report within 48 hours.
- are protected, as good faith reporting is assumed.
- do not have to release their name as part of the school report.
- understand that there is not a statute of limitations on child abuse reporting.

Child abuse and neglect are defined in both state and federal law, and the standard of what constitutes abuse varies from state to state (Child Welfare Information Gateway, 2008c). Professionals can determine what constitutes abuse or neglect in their own state by visiting the "State Statutes Search" Web site at http://www.childwelfare.gov/systemwide/laws_policies/state/can/reporting.cfm.

School counselors are mandated in all states to report suspected abuse under penalty of criminal charges. Some statutes even go as far as to lay out penalties to those who, however misguided or misinformed, do not act accordingly. Certainty is not required; reasonable suspicion, even in the absence of hard evidence, is all the law requires. Mandated reporters are immune from legal proceedings brought by parents or guardians who have been erroneously reported to child protective services. State-specific information about the legal rights and responsibilities of reporters of child abuse, policies, and hotline numbers can be found at http://www.childwelfare.gov/responding/index.cfm (Child Welfare Information Gateway, 2008b). A visit to this Web site can provide extensive information not only about state-specific guidelines, but also about the state-by-state level of incidence for child abuse and neglect.

Good faith reporting is assumed when a professional reports suspected child abuse. A mere suspicion of abuse is all that is necessary to require a report. By reporting his or her suspicions and the observed signs on which those suspicions are based, the professional school counselor has acted legally and ethically. If the report was not made, and it was determined that abuse actually did occur, then legal action could be taken against the school counselor for failing to report. By reporting the suspicion, the school counselor becomes immune from all liability. Each state and territory in the United States provides some form of immunity from liability for persons who, in good faith, report suspected instances of abuse or neglect under local reporting laws. Immunity statutes protect reporters from any civil or criminal liability that they might otherwise incur (Child Welfare Information Gateway, 2008c). Two school counselor/educator-focused articles addressing the legal and ethical issues surrounding child abuse and neglect are helpful as follow up resources for the school counselor to consult (Lambie, 2005; Smith & Lambie, 2005).

Ethical Issues

Often, when a school counselor makes a child abuse report, the parents can easily ascertain by questioning the child who made the report to protective services. If the parents are in conflict with the school counselor over the report, working with the child can be complicated. In many school districts, parents can refuse counseling services for their child even if the student still desires to come in for counseling. Just as teachers may do their job without parental permission, generally speaking, so may school counselors. However, because counseling involves the personal/social/emotional arena, it is considered best practice to have parental permission for individual counseling. When parents have expressly stated that they do not want counseling for their child, it should be a rare exception when the professional school counselor ignores their wishes. Trying to reason with the parents might be beneficial, and if the child needs help, implore them to at least agree to allow someone else to help. Perhaps the parents would allow you to transfer the student's case to another counselor in the school. A counselor does not want to give up easily in an effort to get a student the help he or she needs. Advocacy for the student can sometimes be fulfilled in other ways besides personally delivering the services (Stone, 2005).

If the school counselor still believes that the child is in danger and the parents are trying to conceal their abusive behavior, the counselor is still involved and is required by law to call child protective services.

The case study below is a practical example demonstrating the need for reporting.

These suspicions of possible abuse did not arise in the context of an individual counseling session, a teacher referral, or a student's self-referral but rather through second-hand information from peers. School counselors are cautioned against investigating abuse reports; but, when needed, counselors can ask questions and do some following up, such as talking with Sharone directly or checking with her teachers to see if they have noticed any changes in her. Consulting with the school principal or supervisor of guidance is a good step. It is also appropriate to decide not to ask further questions, but simply make the call to protective services. If the girls who first approached with their suspicions seem credible, and one feels there is reasonable suspicion, then that is enough to

---

Sharone: A School-Based Case Study

Two sixth-grade girls approach their school counselor about a third girl, Sharone. The girls tell the counselor that they believe Sharone's stepfather is sexually molesting her. The girls are vague about details and confused about why they believe their friend is being abused, and they just keep saying that Sharone says "things" that hint at abuse, and they cannot give you any details, only the same very vague statements. They says that their suspicions have been building for months. What is the next step that the school counselor should take?

generate the necessary call to child protective services. If the girls do not appear to be credible, and one does not feel there is reasonable suspicion, it is prudent to follow up with questions of key people such as Sharone or her teacher to make certain something is not being overlooked (Stone, 2005).

Sexual Abuse in Schools

Another instance in which reporting child abuse is essential is teacher-on-student sexual abuse. *Doe v. Rains Independent School District* (1994) was a court case in Texas in which a teacher was involved in a sexual relationship with a student, and another teacher had knowledge of the relationship but waited several months before reporting it. Dana White's student, Sarah Doe, told her that she was having an affair with a teacher at a neighboring school. Sarah told Ms. White that the relationship was hidden under the guise of babysitting. Ms. White did not report the incident at this time because of a promise of confidentiality she made to Sarah. Ms. White continued to talk with Sarah and with other school officials, but did not report Sarah's abuse to proper authorities until weeks later. Once the facts were divulged to the parents of Sarah Doe, they sued Dana White for depriving Sarah of rights granted to her by Texas state law and by the federal constitution. The Texas law that Ms. White allegedly violated was one stating that teachers are required to report child abuse within 48 hours (Stone, 2005). The court found in favor of Dana White. School counselors do not want to find themselves a party to a lawsuit involving the non-report of sexual abuse. Even if the court finds in the professional school counselor's favor, the stress, strain, and emotional toll will be immense, not to mention the realization of the harm caused to a child.

The differentiation in power between a school counselor and a student is considerable, and therefore constitutes a great potential for abuse. School counselors hold influence and sway over vulnerable minors, and though this power is rarely abused, there are school counselors who abuse their position of trust, and although it may or may not be accepted as a reportable offense by child protective services, it is grounds for dismissal.

As reported in *The (Annapolis, MD) Capital* (Capital-Gazette Communications, Inc., "School advisor's dismissal stands," October 19, 2004), a 28-year veteran

---

A School-Based Case Study

A school counselor's colleague does not exercise appropriate professional distance from students. He acts "chummy" with some students and asks them to call him by his first name. He is crossing a line, and you believe he may be involved in dual relationships with students that are harmful. A student of his approaches the school counselor, extremely upset, and tells her that this colleague has asked her about very personal issues, such as whether she is a virgin. He then proceeded to tell her about his sex life. Is this child abuse?

counselor in a Maryland high school was to be dismissed due to inappropriate sexual comments made to students. A county judge upheld this veteran counselor's dismissal for alleged sexual comments made to a female student during a counseling session. Circuit Court Judge David S. Bruce went on to suggest that school counselors should consider asking a third party to attend student interviews when sensitive topics are being discussed. Judge Bruce said that the counselor went well beyond acceptable limits by asking the student about her sex life with her boyfriend, whom the female student complained "treated (her) like crap." Judge Bruce noted that the counselor had a legal obligation to determine if the girl was a victim of sexual abuse, but then stepped way over the limits when he asked her how many times she and her boyfriend had had sex, which sex acts she liked, whether certain sex acts hurt her, and whether she knew any gay or lesbian students in the school. The girl reported the incident to her friend who, in turn, told her mother, who called social services. The social services investigators dismissed the girl's complaint but referred the case to the Board of Education. In 2003, both the local and state boards voted to dismiss the counselor. The counselor's attorney complained that it was the female student's word against his client's, but Judge Bruce said the county judge heard the witnesses and found the girl more credible. The counselor did not face criminal charges in the matter.

PREVENTION AND INTERVENTIONS

Schools are ideal places in which to provide a positive impact on instances of child sexual abuse through prevention programs. School counselors can coordinate or participate in team efforts to build prevention programs that can be used in classroom guidance. Nearly 15 years ago, a majority of school districts were already offering prevention programs (e.g., Daro 1994; Finkelhor & Dziuba-Leatherman, 1995), and they continue to be widespread in the public education system. However, a study of 177 accredited private K–12 schools in Texas revealed that only about 25% of those schools reported using a student-based prevention program. Family involvement, faculty and staff training on child sexual abuse, and program evaluation were lacking (Lanning & Massy-Stokes, 2006). School-initiated sexual abuse prevention programs appear to be largely effective in the United States and abroad (e.g., Davis & Gidycz, 2000; Kenny, Capri, Thakkar-Kolar, Ryan, & Runyon, 2008; Zwi et al., 2007). In these programs, children are generally taught self-protective skills to use when confronted with actual abusive situations, how to recognize and resist improper touching, how to reassure themselves that any sexual abuse was not their fault, and how to learn the correct names for their private parts (Kenny et al.).

Involving parents in the school-based sexual abuse prevention program can actually reduce the prevalence of sexual abuse, given that many of the necessary conditions for abuse are related to family characteristics and the nature of the parent-child bond. Moreover, it is critical that teachers and parents be aware of the tactics typically used by child sexual offenders.

Examples from the University of Calgary's (2002) *School-based Violence Prevention Programs: A Resource Manual* overviewing successful school-based prevention programs are reviewed below (see also Kenny et al., 2008, for a review).

- Child Assault Prevention (CAP; ages 3–18). Developed by the Women Against Rape organization in Columbus, Ohio, this program offers school workshops for children, teachers, and parents led by trained CAP facilitators. Classroom presentations are approximately one hour in length and include information and strategies to assist children and youth in resisting abuse. Abuse is seen as a violation of the children's personal rights. Topics covered include sexual, verbal, emotional, and physical abuse by peers (bullying) and known adults and strangers (abduction). Guided group discussions, narratives, and role-playing activities assist students in learning prevention and protection strategies such as assertiveness, peer support, a self-defense yell, and telling a trusted adult if abuse occurs. Facilitators are trained to handle disclosures. Children can meet individually with a facilitator after the program, if they wish.

- Child Abuse Prevention Program (CAPP; grades K–3, ages 4–8). Five lessons center on five interrelated storybooks entitled *Let's Talk About Touching, Private Parts, Surprises, Tell Someone,* and *Remember.* Each story contains specific rules and behaviors that a child can use if confronted with a potential abuser. Behavior rehearsal during the story and questions in follow-up exercises provide opportunities to practice the skills and concepts presented.

- Body Safety Training (BST; grades K–3, ages 3–7). The emphasis of this program is on developing prevention skills in young children using information and techniques such as modeling, rehearsal, social reinforcement, shaping, and feedback. The classroom teacher, a trained facilitator, or a parent teaches the BST program to small groups of children using a script and picture cards. Groups of four to ten allow each child the time to practice the behavioral skills presented.

- Good Touch/Bad Touch (grades K–6, ages 4–12 years). The primary focus of this program is sexual abuse prevention; however, physical abuse and bullying prevention are included in the Grade 3 program, and sexual harassment and emotional abuse in Grade 5. Children learn five body safety rules, body ownership, how to say "no" to potential abuse, who can help them when abuse does occur, how to ask adults questions about an other adult's behaviors, and that sexual abuse is never a child's fault. Materials and techniques, such as role-playing, reinforce the concepts presented and offer opportunities to practice the skills.

- Red Flag, Green Flag People (grades K–4, elementary-school age). The somewhat dated *Red Flag, Green Flag People* 30-page workbook teaches children about appropriate and inappropriate touches—called "Green Flag" touches and "Red Flag" touches. Role-playing is recommended to reinforce the learned concepts and skills (e.g., recognizing good and bad touches, telling adults if abuse has happened). The facilitator's guide includes objectives, discussion questions, notes, and optional activities, such as role-playing activities to accompany each page of the children's book. In the curriculum version of the program, the children's workbook is a loose-leaf binder that can be photocopied for classroom use. The kindergarten program introduces abuse prevention and teaches prevention skills to groups of children ages 5 and 6. It consists of three 6-minute videotape episodes teaching appropriate and inappropriate touches, how to say "no" to uncomfortable touches, how to get away from abusive situations, and how to identify and tell someone who will help.

- Safe Child (ages 3–10). The program is presented in a preschool through Grade 3 series that includes videos, lesson plans, games, role-playing activities, and other activities for each grade level. The curriculum consists of 5 to 10 lessons per grade level. Videotapes are used to ensure that the concepts and techniques are presented in a consistent way. Video segments are followed by class activities such as role-playing and discussion groups to provide children with structured opportunities for practicing the skills presented. Sexual, emotional, and physical abuse prevention skills are taught in kindergarten, Grade 1, and Grade 3. These lessons include messages such as: "my body belongs to me"; "saying no"; "talking to someone until you receive help"; and "punishment that leaves bruises and marks that are there the next day is excessive". Safety with strangers is covered in preschool and kindergarten. Grades 1 and 2 programs include rules about behaviors when approached by a stranger. Self-care with Grade 2 children explores staying safe in unsupervised situations, such as answering the phone or door, handling free time, and emergency situations. An evaluation form for teachers and school administrators is included in the community-planning guidebook. The form asks for comments about problems or concerns, benefits and positive aspects of the program, children's and parents' reactions, and suggestions for changes to materials or teacher training.

- Preventing Sexual Abuse: Activities and Strategies for Those Working with Children and Adolescents (grades K–12). The curriculum is divided into kindergarten through Grade 6 and Grade 7 through Grade 12. Topics are presented in 1-to-5-day segments depending on the topic and grade level. Curriculum explains ways that children and youth may be tricked into sexual abuse situations, that sexual abuse is not "normal," and that keeping such secrets is not appropriate. Strategies and resources for dealing with sexual abuse, sexual harassment, and sexual assault are presented. Role-playing activities and activity sheets are provided. Information on adapting the materials for the developmentally disabled is in the program manual.

- Kid & Teen SAFE (grades 1–12). Customized presentations are available for children and youth with disabilities who receive special education services. Topics include the differences between okay and not-okay touches, words, and looks; terminology for public and private body parts; personal safety rules and role-playing activities; healthy sexuality; harassment and bullying. SafePlace provides free counseling for persons with disabilities who have been sexually exploited. Counseling promotes healing and provides education to reduce the risk of future abuse.

- No-Go-Tell Protection Curriculum for Young Children with Special Needs (grades K–3). The Lexington Center for the Deaf conducted the research upon which this program was developed and revised. Four fundamental concepts are covered: boundaries with family, friends, familiar people, and strangers; okay and not-okay touches; private body parts and inappropriate touch; and who and how to tell if abuse occurs. The back of the 76 included picture cards each provide information on the concept presented, background information, and suggested activities such as role-playing, stories, and skill-rehearsal strategies.

- Our Children's Future. This 9-lesson curriculum focuses on topics such as personal space, communication and feelings, parts of the body, personal safety, and who can help. Step-by-step instructions and a safe conduct role-playing activity are provided for teachers.

To review, school initiatives can be a viable prevention and intervention tool, but they need to be fully implemented and far more research is need to demonstrate their efficacy. They can help children avoid the development of unhealthy coping mechanisms and the repression of significant memories. When disclosure is encouraged, positive learning can ensue. In short, schools are in an ideal position to help prevent child sexual abuse from occurring by facilitating school-wide prevention programs, such as those listed above, that answer the students' developmental needs.

SUMMARY

School counselors are well situated to promote healthy sexual development in students through their role as consultant, leader, advocate, counselor, and coordinator. A role the school counselor often serves is provider of critical information, bringing awareness to teachers and other educators about normal developmental sexual behavior, symptoms of sexual abuse, and intervention and prevention techniques that help more children develop into happy, healthy, well-adjusted adults. The school counselor as consultant is often the point person in the schools when a report of sexual abuse is required for the child protective services. School counselors can be experts in identifying the signs of abuse and are often called upon to take action, knowing that there is tremendous support for them in the law and in their ethical codes. For additional resources, UCLA's Center for Mental Health in Schools has a Web site, "Gateway to a World of Resources for Enhancing Mental Health" (http://smhp.psych.ucla.edu/gateway/catiiia.htm). It is a clearinghouse of Web links related to child sexual abuse as well as other psychosocial problems.

REFERENCES

American Academy of Child and Adolescent Psychiatry. (2008). *Child sexual abuse.* Retrieved June 4, 2009, from http://www.aacap.org/cs/root/facts_for_families/child_sexual_abuse

American Academy of Pediatrics. (n.d.). *Examples of sexual behaviors in children aged 2 through 6 years.* Retrieved June 3, 2009, from http://www.aap.org/pubserv/PSVpreview/pages/behaviorchart.html

American School Counselor Association. (2003). *The professional school counselor and child abuse and neglect prevention.* Alexandria, VA: Author. Retrieved June 5, 2009, from http://asca2.timberlakepublishing.com//files/PS_Child%20Abuse.pdf

Bancroft, J. (Ed.). (2003). *Sexual development in childhood.* Bloomington, IN: Indiana University Press.

Berliner, L., & Conte, J. R. (1995). The effects of disclosure and intervention on sexually abused children. *Child Abuse & Neglect, 19,* 371–384.

Brown, S. D., Brack, G., & Mullis, F. Y. (2008). Traumatic symptoms in sexually abused children: Implications for school counselors. *Professional School Counseling, 11,* 368–379.

Capital-Gazette Communications, Inc. (October 19, 2004). Annapolis, MD.

Child Welfare Information Gateway. (2007). *Recognizing child abuse and neglect: Signs and symptoms.* Retrieved October 28, 2009, from http://www.childwelfare.gov/pubs/factsheets/signs.cfm

Child Welfare Information Gateway. (2008a). Indicators of child sexual abuse. Retrieved June 3, 2009, from http://www.childwelfare.gov/pubs/usermanuals/sexabuse/sexabusec.cfm

Child Welfare Information Gateway. (2008b). *Responding to child abuse and neglect.* Retrieved October 28, 2009, from http://www.childwelfare.gov/responding/index.cfm

Child Welfare Information Gateway. (2008c). *State laws on reporting and responding to child abuse and neglect.* Retrieved June 3, 2009, from http://www.childwelfare.gov/systemwide/laws_policies/state/can/reporting.cfm

Children's Bureau (US Department of Health and Human Services). (2009a). *Investigation or assessment and victimization rates, 1990–2004 child maltreatment 2004.* Retrieved June 4, 2009, from http://www.acf.hhs.gov/programs/cb/pubs/cm04/figure3_2.htm

Children's Bureau (US Department of Health and Human Services). (2009b). *Summary.* Retrieved June 3, 2009, from http://www.acf.hhs.gov/programs/cb/pubs/cm04/summary.htm

Chromy, S. (2007). Sexually abused children who exhibit sexual behavior problems: Victimization characteristics. *Brief Treatment & Crisis Intervention, 7,* 25–33.

Curry, N. E., & Arnaud, S. H. (1995). Personality difficulties in preschool children as revealed through play themes and styles. *Young Children, 50*(4), 4–9.

Darkness to Light. (2008). *Statistics surrounding child sexual abuse.* Retrieved June 5, 2009, from http://www.darkness2light.org/KnowAbout/statistics_2.asp

Daro, D. A. (1994). Prevention of child sexual abuse. *The Future of Children, 4,* 198–223.

Davis, M. K., & Gidycz, C. A. (2000). Child sexual abuse prevention programs: A meta-analysis. *Journal of Clinical Child Psychology, 29,* 257–265.

DeVoe, E. R., & Faller, K. C. (1999). The characteristics of disclosure among children who may have been sexually abused. *Child Maltreatment, 4,* 217–227.

Doe v. Rains Independent School District 865 F. Supp. 375 (E.D. Tex 1994)

Einbender, A. J., & Friedrich, W. N. (1989). Psychological functioning and behavior of sexually abused girls. *Journal of Consulting and Clinical Psychology, 57,* 155–157.

England, L. W., & Thompson, C. L. (1988). Counseling child sexual abuse victims: Myths and realities. *Journal of Counseling & Development, 66,* 370–373.

Fieldman, J. P., & Crespi, T. D. (2002). Child sexual abuse: Offenders, disclosure, and school-based initiatives. *Adolescence, 37,* 151–161.

Finkelhor, D., & Dziuba-Leatherman, J. (1995). Victimization prevention programs: A national survey of children's exposure and reactions. *Child Abuse & Neglect, 19,* 125–135.

Finkelhor, D., & Jones, L. M. (2004, January). *Explanations for the decline in child sexual abuse cases.* Juvenile Justice Bulletin published by US Department of Justice and Office of Juvenile Justice and Delinquency Prevention (OJJDP), retrieved June 4, 2009, from http://www.ncjrs.gov/pdffiles1/ojjdp/199298.pdf

Gil, E., & Johnson, T. C. (1993). *Sexualized children: Assessment and treatment of sexualized children and children who molest.* Rockville, MD: Launch Press.

Hall, D. K., Matthews, F., & Pearce, J. (1998). Factors associated with sexual behavior problems in young sexually abused children. *Child Abuse and Neglect, 22,* 1045–1063.

Hershkowitz, I. (2009). Socioemotional factors in child sexual abuse investigations. *Child Maltreatment, 14,* 172–181.

James, S. H., & Burch, K. M. (1999). School counselors' roles in cases of child sexual behavior. *Professional School Counseling, 2,* 211–218.

Kelly, R. J. (1993). Effects on sexuality. In J. Waterman, R. J. Kelly, M. K. Oliveri, & J. McCord (Eds.), *Behind the playground walls: Sexual abuse in preschools* (pp. 120–133). New York: Guilford.

Kenny, M. C., Capri, V., Thakkar-Kolar, R. R., Ryan, E. E., & Runyon, M. K. (2008). Child sexual abuse: from prevention to self-protection. *Child Abuse Review, 17,* 36–54.

Korkman, J., Santtila, P., Drzewiecki, T., & Sandnabba, N. (2007). Failing to keep it simple: Language use in child sexual abuse interviews with 3–8-year-old children. *Psychology, Crime & Law, 14,* 41–60.

Lambie, G. W. (2005). Child abuse and neglect: *A practical guide for professional school counselors. Professional School Counseling, 8,* 249–258.

Lanning, B., & Massy-Stokes, M. (2006). Child sexual abuse prevention programs in Texas accredited non-public schools. *American Journal of Health Studies, 21,* 36–43.

London, K., Bruck, M., Ceci, S. J., & Shuman, D. W. (2005). Disclosure of child sexual abuse: What does the research tell us about the ways that children tell? *Psychology, Public Policy, and Law, 11,* 194–226.

Pipe, M-E., & Salmon, K. (2009). Dolls, drawing, body diagrams, and other props: Role of props in investigative interviews. In K. Kuehnle & M. Connell (Eds.), *The evaluation of child sexual abuse allegations: A comprehensive guide to assessment and testimony* (pp. 365–395). Hoboken, NJ: John Wiley.

Sadowski, P. M., & Loesch, L. C. (1993). Using children's drawings to detect potential child sexual abuse. *Elementary School Guidance and Counseling, 28,* 115–123.

University of Calgary School-based Violence Prevention Programs: A Resource Manual. (2002). *Prevention programs addressing child sexual abuse.* Retrieved June 5, 2009, from http://www.ucalgary.ca/resolve/violenceprevention/English/reviewprog/childsxprogs.htm

Sorenson, T., & Snow, B. (1991). How children tell: The process of disclosure in child sexual abuse. *Child Welfare, 70*(1), 3–15.

Smith, T. W., & Lambie, G. W. (2005). Teachers' responsibilities when adolescent abuse and neglect are suspected. *Middle School Journal, 36,* 33–40.

Stone, C. (2005). *School counseling principles: Ethics and law.* Alexandria, VA: American School Counselor Association.

Tillman, K. S. (2004). *Human figure drawings: evaluating trends in child victims of sexual abuse.* Retrieved June 3, 2009, from http://counselingoutfitters.com/vistas/vistas04/21.pdf

White, J., & Allers, C. T. (1994). Play therapy with abused children: A review of the literature. *Journal of Counseling & Development, 72,* 390–394.

Wilder, P. (1991). A counselor's contribution to the child abuse referral network. *The School Counselor, 38,* 203–214.

Zuckerman, E. L. (1993). *The clinician's thesaurus* (3rd ed.). Pittsburgh, PA: The Clinician's Tool Box.

Zwi, K., Woolfenden, S., Wheeler, D. M., O'Brien, T., Tait, P., Williams, K. J. (2007). School-based education programmes for the prevention of child sexual abuse. *Cochrane Database of Systematic Reviews* 2007, Issue 3. Art. No.: CD004380. DOI:10.1002/14651858.CD004380.pub2. Retrieved June 5, 2009, from http://mrw.interscience.wiley.com/cochrane/clsysrev/articles/CD004380/frame.html

Chapter 7

Students with Severe Acting-Out Behavior

A Family Intervention Approach

KEITH M. DAVIS

Appalachian State University

Highly disruptive behavior is a challenging problem to deal with effectively in a school setting. Of course, professional school counselors will attempt to use the systems approach (e.g., Hawe, Shiell, & Riley, 2009), where they work within multiple contexts in an attempt to support the troubled student. Perhaps due to time constraints or a lack of training, the family system is often neglected in this approach. It is, however, important for the school counselor who is operating out of a comprehensive school counseling program to use strengths-based, time-limited family interventions (American School Counselor Association, 2005). Most school counselors agree that involving families in their children's educations has a significant positive impact on the academic, personal/social, and career aspirations of students. When families are actively engaged in their children's academic, personal/social, and career activities, there is a higher likelihood that the educational experience will have a positive outcome (Amatea, Daniels, Bringman, & Vandiver, 2004; Amatea, Smith-Adcock, & Villares, 2006; Davis, 2001; Davis & Lambie, 2005; Duhon & Manson; 2000; Galassi & Akos, 2007; Ravthvon, 2008; Reink, Splett, Robeson, & Offutt, 2008; Thomas & Ray, 2006).

This chapter is intended to supplement the earlier chapter on externalizing behavior problems by first providing a real-life school-based case study of how a high school counselor intervened with a youth who was severely acting out (disruptive behavior) in the school by assisting the family. Then the essential characteristics of acting-out behaviors, often classified as a "behavior disorder (BD)" in the school setting, are overviewed. Third, key research-based family interventions employed by the professional school counselor are discussed. Finally, the chapter provides additional resources that can be used by practicing professional school counselors and counselors-in-training to assist students and families with behavioral challenges.

David's case may sound familiar to many professional school counselors, who often work with children and adolescents who present with severe acting-out behaviors. A brief overview of the essential characteristics of acting-out behaviors in children and adolescents will help professional school counselors in their work.

David: A School-Based Case Study

David was a 15-year-old white male freshman in high school who was referred to his high school counselor as a result of frequent physical fights (resulting in suspensions from school), school attendance and truancy issues, and using foul language to teachers. Despite having no identified learning disabilities and a record of successful academic achievement in elementary and middle school, David was failing several classes. David's grades and conduct began to come into question during Grade 7, and continued until his current referral.

David was identified by others, including the high school counselor, as an angry and aggressive teenager. He was clearly not pleased to be speaking with the school counselor. As a result it took several meetings for the counselor to establish a positive rapport with David and help him realize that the meetings were not punishment, but a genuine attempt to understand him and his worldview. When asked his thoughts on why things began to turn for the worse during middle school, David could offer no answer other than: "Everybody is against me and I don't take no crap from anyone." When asked about his family, David reported that he was an only child, his mother worked part-time, and his father was a truck driver, who was gone several days a week on long hauls. David seemed indifferent when the counselor asked if it was all right with him to have his parents to come in for a meeting.

When phoned, David's mother agreed to come in for a meeting with the school counselor, but said it might not be possible for David's father as he was frequently gone for his job. Meeting with David's mother only at first, the counselor confirmed that David had not been in any trouble before seventh grade. When asked what had changed during that time, David's mother noted that it seemed to have begun when David's father was laid off from his factory job, was out of work for a couple of months until he took the truck driving job, and was then gone most of the time. David had become less manageable during this time, and was frequently left alone while his mother worked part time.

ESSENTIAL CHARACTERISTICS OF ACTING-OUT BEHAVIORS

This section briefly discusses several characteristics of acting-out behaviors as defined by the *Diagnostic and Statistical Manual of Mental Disorders, Fourth Edition, Text Revision*, also known as the DSM–IV–TR (American Psychiatric Association [APA], 2000). For a comprehensive understanding of the complete diagnostic criteria for acting-out behaviors most commonly experienced in childhood and adolescence (e.g., Attention-Deficit/Hyperactivity Disorder; Conduct Disorder; and Oppositional Defiant Disorder), a reading of pages 85–102 in the DSM–IV–TR is recommended (see also Chapter 2).

Common Diagnostic Features and Associated Factors

The prevalence of acting-out behaviors has increased over the years and is often diagnosed more in urban settings than rural. Although behavioral symptoms vary with age, behaviors tend to escalate in severity as the individual develops "increased physical strength, cognitive abilities, and sexual maturity" (APA, 2000, p. 97). Males outnumber females in the diagnosis, and differences between the genders demonstrate that males tend to exhibit more acting-out behaviors associated with physical confrontations and property vandalism, while females tend to exhibit more behaviors associated with lying, truancy, running away, substance abuse, and prostitution. Children and adolescents who act out may also experience "low frustration tolerance, temper outbursts, bossiness, stubbornness, excessive and frequent insistence that requests be met, mood swings, demoralization, dysphoria, rejection by peers, and poor self-esteem" (APA, p. 88). Finally, there are often "conflicts with parents, teachers, and peers" (APA, p. 100) that develop as a result of the behaviors.

Caution should be taken when assuming acting-out behavior diagnoses for children or adolescents who immigrate to the United States from war-ravaged countries, or areas of the United States where crime or poverty are widespread. Adverse behaviors in these children and adolescents may be outgrowths of protective behaviors developed in their sociocultural context.

In David's case, his acting-out behavior diagnosis was made based on information from his teachers and school administrators, his former middle school counselor, by meeting with his mother, and the school counselor's observations of and discussions with David himself. Specifically in David's case, he exhibited repetitive and persistent acting-out behaviors, such as fighting, intimidation and bullying, breaking in and destruction of personal property, stealing, staying out at night, running away from home, and truancy/attendance issues at school. These behaviors had caused significant impairment to David's social and academic functioning. For David, there was no documentation that any of these behaviors existed before the age of 10. His troubled behavior began in seventh grade when he was 13 years old, and interestingly enough, shortly after his father lost his factory job and began working as a long-haul truck driver. This led the school counselor to think systemically about David and his family, and conclude that a family intervention was warranted.

EFFECTIVE FAMILY INTERVENTIONS

The fact that David's behavior began to deteriorate at about the same time his father lost his job and subsequently took on work truck driving, requiring him to be away from the home several days at a time, was too coincidental. Immediately, the school counselor began forming a systems perspective for understanding David and his behavior.

A family systems perspective attempts to understand individual human behavior within an interrelated social and familial context (Amatea et al., 2006; Davis, 2001; Duhon & Manson; 2000; Fine, 1992; Fine & Carlson, 1992; Hawe et al., 2009; Hinkle, 1993; Hinkle & Wells, 1995; Reink et al., 2008). School-age children and adolescents belong to several systems (e.g., family, school, community, and cultural), all of which combine and interrelate to form a series of subsystems within one larger system. Thus, when professional school counselors consider problem behaviors in school-age children and adolescents, the outlook from a family systems perspective is that these problem behaviors may result from dysfunctional family interactions, rather than placing blame for the problem behaviors on the child alone (Hinkle & Wells, 1995). In these cases school counselors should want to switch from a deficits approach to a strengths-based, family resiliency perspective (Amatea et al.; Galassi & Akos, 2007).

Specific Family Interventions

Examples of positive family interventions employed by professional school counselors within the school have received increasing attention in the school-counseling literature. Briefly described below are several examples of family interventions that can be employed in a school setting by professional school counselors, concluding with a more comprehensive description of the case study presented earlier in the chapter.

Collaborative and Systemic Consultation   Mirroring in several ways Dinkmeyer and Carlson's (2006) processes, Amatea et al. (2004) discussed a four-step collaborative consultation process that could be employed as a way to facilitate stronger home-school relations and encourage family engagement in their children's education.

- *Step 1. Assessment.* The first step involves school counselors assessing the initial attitudes and practices of all school personnel relative to all family-school communications.

- *Step 2. Education.* This phase involves the education of school personnel, with school counselors modeling the collaborative process for all school personnel. School counselors accomplish this by seeking input from all school personnel in a such a way that hinders "the blaming that undermines many family-school problem-solving routines and engages in joint problem solving" (Amatea et al., pp. 50–51). This step also includes opportunities for school counselors to arrange meetings with teachers, families, and students in an effort for all parties to become active participants in school-based decisions, with emphasis placed on a no-fault, co–decision-making model for educational success.

- *Step 3. Restructuring.* This step examines family-school interaction patterns, revising the manner in which family-school meetings are traditionally conducted. By collaborating with teachers, school counselors are able to establish biweekly grade-level meetings in which families are invited to join with their children in non-problematic and student/family-led conferences for educational decision-making.

- *Step 4. Evaluation and accommodation.* Finally, this step allows school counselors to elicit feedback from students, families, and school personnel regarding the overall effectiveness of the collaborative and systemic approach.

Imaginative-Constructivist Model   This strengths-based approach for family intervention integrates concepts from narrative and solution-focused therapies (de Shazer, 1985; Eppler, Olsen, & Hidano, 2009; Freeman, Epston, & Lobovits, 1997) with school counseling activities and services (Galassi & Akos, 2007). Narrative approaches help families change how they view their current circumstances by restructuring how they tell their personal stories. Solution-focused strategies help families focus on current strengths (i.e., what is already working for the family), exceptions to the problem (i.e., times when the problem is not happening), and what the family would want ideally to happen (Eppler et al.). Thomas and Ray (2006) provide excellent examples of this intervention approach in their work with the families of gifted children, children with learning disabilities, and children with behavior problems. Their two-phase intervention is comprised of an assessment phase followed by a phase during which intervention techniques are implemented.

- *Phase 1. Assessment.* An informal assessment by the school counselor is conducted, using information gathered from family interviews and from listening to "the stories each family member brings to the session" (Thomas & Ray, 2006, p. 62).

- *Phase 2. Implementation.* The school counselor uses a narrative approach to help the family restructure their personal stories. Having families restructure their stories facilitates the change process "because changing the stories people tell about themselves and others changes their situation" (Thomas & Ray, 2006, p. 62). A tool for facilitating the restructuring of family stories involves moving from "thin descriptions" of family lives, which tend to be more stereotypical and rigid, to more complex "thick descriptions," which encompass multiple perspectives (Geertz, 2000; White & Epston, 1990).

In describing their work with families of gifted children, Thomas and Ray (2006) stated, "A typical thin description of giftedness primarily presents the benefits of being gifted. A thick description also would talk about the drawbacks of being gifted" (p. 62). Some specific questions put forth by these authors for school counselors were "How does the giftedness of one person affect the family and the school? Who has a vested interest in the giftedness of this person? What does giftedness do for the family?" (p. 62).

To support a family with a child who is acting out, sample questions based within a solution-focused orientation might include "How is the trouble your child is getting in to working for this family? Was there a time when your child's behavior was not a concern (i.e., exceptions to the problem; times when the problem was not happening)? What would the family ideally like to see happen with this acting-out behavior?" With solution-focused family interventions, the main goal of the school counselor is to focus the family on times when the family was already successful and encourage them to reproduce those times, re-enacting what exactly had to happen to pave the way the for those successes.

Time-Limited Structural-Strategic Family Counseling Interventions   The landmark book written by Hinkle and Wells (1995) detailed how professional school counselors can employ a family systems perspective in schools, what training school counselors can receive in family counseling and interventions, and specific techniques that have been proven in a school environment. The book also contains a variety of case studies looking at the ways in which practicing professional school counselors were able to successfully employ time-limited family counseling and interventions in their individual schools. As a further example, Davis (2001) described a family counseling intervention he employed while working as an elementary school counselor. This family intervention used a structural and strategic approach to reestablish a shared parental subsystem between the grandmother and mother of an elementary-school-age child who was exhibiting increasingly aggressive behavior at school as a result of a conflicted parental subsystem.

Structural-Strategic Family Intervention

Both structural and strategic interventions help families see how their patterns of interacting with one another might contribute to dysfunction within the family, which often might be expressed in behavioral and learning challenges suffered at school by children and adolescents (Davis, 2001; Hinkle & Wells, 1995; Thomas & Ray, 2006). Developed by Minuchin (1974), structural family interventions are directed at changing the organization of a family by altering familial interaction patterns. Family structure refers to the organized ways in which families interact, behavior patterns being typically influenced by a set of rules for each behavior. Within each family there is a structure, with adults and children having differing degrees of authority and influence. In most families, the parents, parent, or guardian typically has authority, responsibility, and influence over the children. A fundamental goal of structural family intervention is to aid the family in solving its own problems by reorganizing the family structure. For example, the school counselor might help the family create a more effective structure, one that typically expects the parent(s) or guardian(s) to be in charge of the whole family, including the children, not the other way around, with children controlling the family through their behaviors.

In strategic family intervention (Haley, 1980; Madanes, 1981, 1984, 1990), a school counselor might employ techniques (e.g., strategies and/or directives) to help families change their thinking, behaviors, and interactions with one another. Strategies and directives are designed to aid the reorganization of family structure. Strategic interventions introduce new behaviors into familial interactions, allowing families to practice these new behaviors between family meetings. Through the practice of the new behaviors, the family can change the existing behavior patterns and interactions that have maintained the dysfunctional behaviors within the family.

In the case study of David and his parents, the school counselor decided to test, through a series of family meetings, a modified structural and strategic intervention. The goal was to help David's parents learn a common parenting strategy in order to support their child.

David's deterioration in academic achievement and social behavior first began in middle school, shortly after his father changed jobs and became "absent" from the family. David's mother was left the task of being "the parent" on her own. When David's father was at home, he was "too tired" from his work to be involved with the family and became disengaged as both a husband and a father (a dysfunctional family interaction pattern). As David's behavior began to deteriorate, his father became even more disengaged. From a family systems perspective, and specifically from a structural family perspective, David no longer felt his parents were on the same page in parenting him. The task for the school counselor was to find a way for David's parents to begin parenting him together again. To facilitate this process, a strategic intervention (i.e., a directive) was offered as a way to bring David's parents together.

Meeting with the parents first, without David, helped begin the process of establishing the parents as "in charge" (i.e., a strategic intervention). The school counselor learned, in talking with the parents, how difficult the transition had been when David's father lost his job and was out of work for two months, and how David's mother, who previously had not worked outside the home, had to begin working in order to support the family. According to David's father, this was difficult in the sense that he himself had been raised with the belief that men were supposed to be the provider for the family. When the job for a long-haul truck driver became available, he immediately took it in order to once again be a provider. David's mother continued to work, as bills had accumulated during the period of David's father's unemployment. Before the job transition took place, the family had been spending a lot of time together, going to the movies together, having backyard barbeques, being involved in Little League baseball, and taking family vacations. With the father often on the road and away from home for long periods, the family was spending less quality family time together. When David's father was on the road, he rarely called home, and when he did, he spoke only to David's mother, and not to David himself. As David's behavior began to deteriorate, phone calls from the road effectively ceased, as conversations between the parents led only to arguments about David and his behavior (i.e., a dysfunctional interaction pattern).

In parallel conversations with David only, the school counselor learned that he felt his father did not care about him anymore, that his father was always gone, and when his father was home, "he didn't give a damn about me." In David's eyes, he did not have a father anymore. In fact, he felt like he did not have a family anymore. David became angry, and this anger resulted in numerous fights at school, school suspensions, staying out late, and eventually legal troubles from breaking and entering and vandalizing homes and property. David also demonstrated contempt for authority figures, mainly his mother and teachers at school, through his use of profanity and defying any direction.

Conceptualizing David and his family, the school counselor did not see David's behavior problems as resting with him alone, but rather the whole family having not successfully adjusted to the father's new work schedule. David's father was disengaged from the rest of the family, the mother exasperated by circumstances, and David feeling like he had no father or family, or authority figure to provide structure. Thus, David's acting-out behavior was a result of dysfunctional family interaction patterns.

Meeting with the parents began the process of reestablishing the parents as parental figures. The strategic directive that was first given in a meeting with the parents was for the father to call home each night when he was on the road. Conversations between the parents during these calls were not to be about David's behavior, with the idea that no arguments about the behavior could therefore take place. Equally important, these phone calls each night would also include a conversation between David and his father as well, to see how David's day went at school and see how he was doing, something that had not previously taken place. This strategic directive would begin a change process in the family's behavior and interactions and divert them from the current dysfunctional pattern.

A second strategic directive given was to not only affirm that the parents for each working hard to provide for David and the family, but that they also deserved quality time together with David, as well as quality time together as husband and wife. By affirming David's father for being a hard worker and provider and acknowledging his being tired when he was home, and acknowledging David's mother as enduring the hardships of having the father absent part of the week, the counselor was able to have them agree to try to spend a little more quality time together as a family and separately as a couple when the father was home.

After speaking with David's parents together, and then David separately, it was time to bring the entire family together to discuss the plan. This served the purpose of bringing the family together as a total family unit. The school counselor was able to obtain agreement from the whole family as a unit that they would try this new pattern of behavior. It was also agreed that as David's academic and social behavior improved, his father would allow David to accompany him on the road with the truck when David did not have school (the third strategic directive). This prospect excited David, as he had expressed an interest in truck driving as part of his future. Subsequent meetings resulted in an agreement that David's father would accompany the family to court to help resolve David's legal troubles for breaking and entering. To further bolster and reinforce the family in change, a family meeting was scheduled at the school with David's teachers and the school principal to help provide support and consistency.

The school counselor met with David's parents together twice monthly after school for about four months to check on progress and provide support, bringing David in to join them at the end of the meetings. The counselor met with David individually on a weekly basis to check up on his academic progress, work on his anger, and reinforce the changes that were taking place. This family had made a commitment with continued support from the counselor, as well as support and understanding from teachers and the school administration. As David's family slowly began to spend more quality together, the father became more engaged in the family and David's behavior began to slowly change for the better. There were a few relapses with continued fights at school; however, all were able to process those relapses in follow-up meetings with the idea that change is a process. The counselor was able to secure from David and his teachers that when he felt like a fight was going to happen, he could immediately come to the counselor's office, or the counseling suite, to sit and "cool off" without question. By the end of the year, David had not been in a fight for the last two months of the school year.

For this case study, it would have been easy to place all the responsibility for his acting-out behavior on David. However, from a family systems perspective, the case can be seen as the family's inability to adjust to changing family circumstance, warranting an intervention at the family level. It is critically important in such cases to not place blame on the parents for their child's misfortune. David certainly had individual responsibility in his behavior choices. At the same time, professional school counselors need to be cognizant and sensitive to changing family circumstances and how these circumstances affect the family and the child, as well as the academic, personal/social, and career aspirations of the child.

RESOURCES FOR PROFESSIONAL
SCHOOL COUNSELORS

For many professional school counselors, the thought of providing family interventions within a school context seems daunting. Many school counselors feel ill prepared or have not received any training to provide such services. With so many demands and responsibilities already placed on professional school counselors, many may not feel they have the additional time to provide such services. In this section there are some suggestions to address these legitimate concerns.

For professional school counselors who may have an interest in providing time-limited family counseling and interventions with the families of school-age children, but feel unprepared to do so, several options are available. Many state, regional, and national school counseling associations provide training in family counseling and interventions, typically at school counseling conferences. Being a member of professional organizations and associations can keep practicing school counselors abreast of presentations, trainings, and opportunities to further their knowledge and skills on a variety of topics germane to the development of the profession. Furthermore, as members of professional organizations and associations, professional school counselors typically receive professional journals and newsletters (both paper and electronic) that share the latest research and proven techniques in the counseling field. At the time of this writing, as a result of being a member of the American School Counselor Association (ASCA), the author received an electronic invitation from ASCA to attend a local training on solution-focused brief counseling and parent consultation.

Another professional association for school counselors to consider, as it relates to increasing knowledge of family counseling and interventions, is the International Association of Marriage and Family Counselors (IAMFC), a subdivision of the American Counseling Association. By being members of IAMFC, professional school counselors to receive *The Family Journal*, a professional journal that publishes the latest research, techniques, and interventions in marriage and family counseling. More information on IAMFC can be found at their Web site: http://www.iamfc.com/index.html.

Another way for professional school counselors to receive training and/or supervision in family counseling and intervention knowledge and skills is through in-service training at the school or school system level. Professional school counselors acting as counselor educators visit several school-system-wide school counselor meetings to provide training and supervision in family counseling and interventions. Many school systems are located near universities that house counselor training programs. Contacting a university counseling program to inquire about providing training and supervision to school counselors in the area is often well received, and an opportunity for the counselor educator to provide a valuable service. Equally, many counseling programs allow already trained school counselors to take courses in marriage and family counseling as a way to stay updated on changes in the profession with further training in knowledge, skills, and supervision. Finally, there is already a strong literature base of professionally published articles and books regarding family interventions employed by professional school counselors. Some are listed in the references here, and are strongly recommended readings.

Some professional school counselors may wonder how in the world they are going to find the time to incorporate family counseling and interventions within the school into already demanding schedules and responsibilities. What works for some is to first realize that any such intervention would be time-limited. Secondly, given all the counselor's other responsibilities, they have to pick and choose which families to work with based on the probability of a successful outcome given the time limitations. For families that need long-term, in-depth psychotherapy, referrals were given to local mental health professionals, with school support coordinated by the school counselor. For families that a school counselor feels could benefit from time-limited counseling and interventions, it can be helpful to work with them at the school, typically after school hours. The school counselor may also be able to negotiate with the school principal for one day a week of flex-time, when the counselor can come into the school at noon and stay well into the evening, seeing up to four families in the afternoon and evening. This also speaks to the importance of having administrative support, so the school counselor can have every opportunity to help students and their families.

SUMMARY

School-age children and adolescents belong to several subsystems, including their school community and family. It is a natural fit to bring these two systems together in the form of time-limited family counseling and interventions within the school. Bringing the family into the school setting and asking them to be part of solution may seem to be just another thing to do on the counselor's agenda, but neglecting this potential source of resiliency and support may in the long run increase the amount of time the counselor spends on students with difficult problems. Research suggests that for some learners who exhibit acting-out behaviors and externalizing disorders in school, supporting them from a family systems perspective increases the likelihood that these students' long-range developmental academic, personal/social, and career goals will be achieved.

REFERENCES

Amatea, E. S., Daniels, H., Bringman, N., & Vandiver, F. M. (2004). Strengthening counselor-teacher-family connections: The family-school collaborative consultation project. *Professional School Counseling*, *8*, 47–55.

Amatea, Smith-Adcock, & Villares, (2006). From family deficit to family strength: Viewing families' contributions to children's learning from a family resilience perspective. *Professional School Counseling*, *9*, 177–189.

American Psychiatric Association. (2000). *Diagnostic and statistical manual of mental disorders* (4th ed., Text Revision). Washington DC: American Psychiatric Association.

American School Counselor Association. (2005). *The professional school counselor and comprehensive school counseling programs*. Retrieved June 6, 2009, from http://asca2.timberlakepublishing.com//files/PS_Comprehensive.pdf

Davis, K. M. (2001). Structural-strategic family counseling: A case study in elementary school counseling. *Professional School Counseling*, *3*, 180–186.

Davis, K. M., & Lambie, G. W. (2005). Family engagement: A collaborative, systemic approach for middle school counselors. *Professional School Counseling*, *9*, 144–151.

de Shazer, S. (1985). *Keys to solution in brief therapy*. New York: W.W. Norton.

Dinkmeyer, D. Jr., & Carlson, J. (2006). *Consultation: Creating school-based interventions* (3rd ed.). New York: Routledge/Taylor & Francis.

Duhon, G. M., & Manson, T. J. (2000). *Preparation, collaboration, and emphasis on the family in school counseling for the new millennium*. New York: Mellen Press.

Eppler, C., Olsen, J. A., & Hidano, L. (2009). Using stories in elementary school counseling: brief, narrative techniques. *Professional School Counseling*, *12*, 387–391.

Fine, M. J. (1992). A systems–ecological perspective on home-school intervention. In M.J. Fine & C. Carlson (Eds.), *The handbook of family-school interventions: A systemic perspective* (pp. 1–17). Needham Heights, MA: Allyn & Bacon.

Fine, M. J., & Carlson, C. (Eds.) (1992). *The handbook of family-school interventions: A systemic perspective.* Needham Heights, MA: Allyn & Bacon.

Freeman, J., Epston, D., & Lobovits, D. (1997). *Playful approaches to serious problems: Narrative therapy with children and their families.* New York: W.W. Norton.

Galassi, J. P., & Akos, P. (2007). *Strengths-based school counseling: Promoting student development and achievement.* New York: Lawrence Erlbaum.

Geertz, C. (2000). Thick description: Toward an interpretive theory of cultures. In C. Geertz (Ed.), *The interpretation of cultures* (pp. 3–32). New York: Harper Collins.

Haley, J. (1980). *Leaving home.* New York: McGraw-Hill.

Hawe, P., Shiell, A., & Riley, T. (2009). Theorising interventions as events in systems. *American Journal of Community Psychology, 43,* 267–276.

Hinkle, J. S. (1993). Training school counselors to do family counseling. *Elementary School Guidance and Counseling, 27,* 252–257.

Hinkle, J. S., & Wells, M. E. (1995). *Family counseling in the schools: Effective strategies and interventions for counselors, psychologists, and therapists.* Greensboro, NC: ERIC/CASS.

Madanes, C. (1981). *Strategic family therapy.* San Francisco, CA: Jossey-Bass.

Madanes, C. (1984). *Behind the one-way mirror: Advances in the practice of strategic therapy.* San Francisco, CA: Jossey-Bass.

Madanes, C. (1990). *Sex, love, and violence.* New York: W. W. Norton.

Minuchin, S. (1974). *Families and family therapy.* Cambridge, MA: Harvard University.

Rathvon, N. (2008). *Effective school interventions: Evidence-based strategies for improving student outcomes* (2nd ed.). New York: Guilford Press.

Reink, W., Splett, J., Robeson, E., & Offutt, C. (2008). Combining school and family interventions for the prevention and early intervention of disruptive behavior problems in children: A public health perspective, *Psychology in the Schools, 46,* 33–43.

Thomas, V., & Ray, K. E. (2006). Counseling exceptional individuals and their families: A systems perspective. *Professional School Counseling, 10,* 58–65.

White, D., & Epston, D. (1990). *Narrative means to therapeutic ends.* New York: W.W. Norton.

Chapter 8

Suicide Issues

JILL PACKMAN AND CATEY BARBER

University of Nevada, Reno,
O'Brien Middle School, Reno, NV

For most professional school counselors there is no mental health issue more devastating than student suicide. Although there are a host of relevant publications, Web sites, and self-help tools, suicidal ideations, actual suicide attempts, and completed suicides continue unabated in schools and society. What makes school-based prevention and intervention so challenging to implement at the local level is the lack of current and accurate statistical information about suicide and related issues.

Incidents of student suicidal ideations and completed suicides are often shrouded by secrecy due, in part, to a misunderstanding of the complex nature of suicidology, public stigma, and the need for confidentiality. From the 1950s to the 1990s, school counselors witnessed a threefold increase in the number of documented suicide attempts (Prinstein, Boergers, Spirito, Little, & Grapentine, 2000), and, sadly, suicide remains a leading cause of death for older children and adolescents (Leslie, Stein, & Rotheram-Borees, 2002; National Institute of Mental Health [NIMH], 2009b).

Given the problem's impact on the various student systems and its multifaceted character, school counselors and school psychologists at all levels are clearly an important resource in the process of preventing suicide, identifying students at risk, and providing ongoing support and care to students, educators, and families (Hull, 2009). This chapter's primary aim is to offer school counselors vital information on this issue with the intention that it can increase their effectiveness in assisting students, families, and other educators in understanding and preventing

Megan: A School-Based Case Study

Every semester the counseling staff at a suburban secondary school sends out a list of peer groups that are starting up, asking students if they would like to participate. This particular spring semester, a particular school counselor was facilitating the self-esteem group. Many students indicated interest in the group. The interested students were screened and the appropriate students were assigned to each group.

In this particular group there were eight students. Things were going well. The students were making connections and working on their perceptions of themselves. During the fifth meeting, group members did an activity that was designed to help the students see how they were perceived by others in contrast to how they perceived themselves. Each student was asked to write his or her name in the center of a piece of paper and draw a vertical line down the paper about an inch from the edge. Near their name inside the border, the students were asked to write words to describe how they saw themselves. When this was complete, the students put their papers in the middle of the group table, picked out another student's paper, and on the outside of the border wrote words to describe how they saw the student whose name was in the middle of the paper. Each student made a comment on every other student's page.

As the school counselor was monitoring the activity, she noticed a word on one student's paper that concerned her: Megan had described herself as "suicidal." Not wanting to call attention to this in the group setting, after the counselor and students processed the activity the counselor asked Megan to stay after the meeting. The counselor let Megan know that she had seen what she had written, and wanted to check in with her. The counselor asked if Megan was thinking of killing herself and she said, "Yes." The counselor also asked if Megan had a plan. She did; she would take her mother's sleeping pills and slit her wrist. She pulled up her sleeves to show the counselor that she had been "practicing." She had slice marks on her wrists near her hands. She stated that she did not see another way out of her current situation and had been feeling badly about herself for some time. She was sad, and things seemed to be getting worse rather than better. When the counselor asked her what would happen if she were to go home after school that day, Megan said she could not promise that she would not attempt to take her own life.

Given Megan's responses, her depressed state, lack of hope, her plan, and her inability to make a promise that she would not attempt suicide, the counselor contacted Megan's parents immediately. Because Megan's mother worked swing shift, it took repeated calls for the counselor to get in touch with her. When the counselor finally reached her, Megan's mother came up to the school immediately so they could discuss the severity of her daughter's suicidal tendencies. Megan was scared to face her mother and worried that she would be angry with her. With the counselor's support, Megan told her mother all the things that had been bothering her, such as the deterioration she perceived in her relationships with friends, fighting with siblings, feeling misunderstood by both family and friends, and feeling disconnected from her parents. Megan's mother responded caringly, saying that she wanted to do what was best for her daughter. Following the policies of both the school and counseling department, Megan's mother immediately took her daughter to the emergency room at the local hospital, where another evaluation was conducted. The medical staff at the emergency room determined that Megan was a threat to herself and placed her in an in-patient treatment program, where she remained for two weeks.

student suicides. After considering a case study, salient background information associated with this mental health concern is overviewed. Before concluding, the chapter discusses practical school counseling-based suggestions for assessment, prevention, intervention, and postvention.

BACKGROUND INFORMATION

Although the data reported below are as current as possible and from highly reputable sources, school counselors should know that these are merely trends and averages; statistics change from year to year, and do not necessarily represent every community and student body. Also, from the fact sheets published, for instance, by the Center for Disease Control and Prevention (2006), it is difficult to tease out the numbers of students who have suicidal *ideations* (self-reported thoughts of suicide-related behavior), who have *threatened* suicide (verbally or nonverbally), and who have *attempted* suicide (self-inflicted harm with or without resulting injuries).

Prevalence

After almost a decade of slight decline (1996–2003), suicide rates among children and youth ages 10 to 19 are again on the rise (Bridge, Greenhouse, & Weldon, 2008). The American Association of Suicidology (AAS; 2008) reported that in 2005, 270 children between the ages of 10 and 14 committed suicide, and 4,212 adolescents between the ages of 15 and 24 ended their own lives. These grim findings correspond with those presented by the National Center for Injury Prevention and Control (2008), stating that youth suicide results in roughly 4,500 deaths each year, with the top three methods employed are firearms (46%), suffocation (39%), and self-poisoning (8%).

In 2004, suicide was the third leading cause of death among adolescents ages 15 to 19 (AAS, 2008), with females far more likely than males in the age group to die by self-inflicted harm (NIMH, 2009b). The 2004 prevalence rates, aggregated by ethnicity, show that non-Hispanic White European Americans and Native Americans have the highest rates of suicide (about 12.7 deaths per 100,000 persons), even as African Americans, Asian/Pacific Islander Americans, and Hispanics have the lowest rates (about 5.7 deaths per 100,000 persons). From these trends, school counselors can see the importance of considering both gender and ethnicity in preventing and intervening with children and youth.

Other pertinent details from the 2004 suicide rates are as follows:

- For children ages 10 to 14, the prevalence rate was 1.3 deaths per 100,000.
- For adolescents ages 15 to 19, the rate was 8.2 deaths per 100,000
- For young adults ages 20 to 24, the rate was 12.5 deaths per 100,000 (NIMH, 2009b).

By 2006, the suicide rate among adolescents had risen slightly to 9.9 deaths per 100,000 (McIntosh, 2009). Medical intervention, however, does appear to influence the adolescent suicide rate. From 1990 to 2000, the teen rate declined somewhat in regions of the United States where treatment using antidepressant medication was the most common (Olfson, Shaffer, Marcus, & Greenberg, 2003).

Looking at data related to suicide attempts (completed or not), we see that for every two or three attempts by adolescent females, there is one attempt by an adolescent male (American Association for Suicidology, 1998; Riesch, Jacobson, Sawdey, Anderson, & Henriques, 2008). Adolescent girls from Hispanic and Latino backgrounds are the most likely to report a suicide attempt (Riesch et al.). The data also show that 1 in 10 girls and 1 in 25 boys will make a suicide attempt at some point in their youth (Esposito & Clum, 2003). Furthermore, 14% of males and 25% of females in high school have seriously considered suicide. Of those, 11% of males and 18% of females had made a specific plan (Savin-Williams & Ream, 2003). It has also been found that girls who have suicidal ideation are more likely to suffer from health problems, to have received psychiatric care, and to have been sexually abused. Boys tend to have more conduct disorders, substance abuse problems, and deviant behaviors (Leslie et al., 2002). Riesch et al. reported a chilling statistic: 18% of sixth-graders have had thoughts of killing themselves.

Warning Signs and Characteristics of Suicide

Being able to identify the warning signs and characteristics of suicidal ideation in a school setting is key to prevention. Before exploring the warning signs and the other related dimensions of suicide, these signs are listed below.

- Observable signs of serious depression:

  Unrelenting low mood

  Pessimism

  Hopelessness

  Desperation

  Anxiety, psychic pain, and inner tension

  Withdrawal

  Sleep problems

  Increased alcohol or other drug use

  Recent impulsiveness and taking unnecessary risks

  Threatening suicide or expressing a strong wish to die

- Making a plan:

  Giving away prized possessions

  Sudden or impulsive purchase of a firearm

  Obtaining other means of killing oneself, such as poisons or medications

- Unexpected rage or anger. (American Foundation for Suicide Prevention [AFSP], 2009c)

Suicide and Mood Disorders   From the above signs, *mood disorders* (usually depression; see Chapter 3 for a detailed discussion) tend to affect a majority of the children and adolescents who commit suicide. Because a clinical diagnosis of a mood disorder is a powerful predicator of suicidal ideation and future suicide completions, school counselors must recognize these signs and symptoms (Caballero & Nahata, 2005) in their students as well.

Two of the most common mood disorders are depression and bipolar disorder (National Mental Health Information Center, 2006). Adolescents with mood disorders are 27 times more likely to complete suicide than those without. The risk of suicide increases when there are coexisting mental disorders (e.g., mood disorder and anxiety, or disruptive behavior and substance abuse; Esposito & Clum, 2003; Riesch et al., 2008). Adolescents with internalizing disorders such as depression exhibit significantly higher levels of suicidal ideation when under high levels of stress (Esposito & Clum).

Moreover, severe depression is a leading cause of suicide *re*-attempts in adolescents. The severity of the depression is a prominent factor in predicting future suicide attempts (Riesch et al., 2008). According to the American Psychiatric Association's *Diagnostic Statistical Manual* (DSM–IV–TR, 2000), depression may exist if the following signs have been present for more than two weeks: poor performance in school, withdrawal from friends and activities, sadness and hopelessness, lack of enthusiasm, energy, or motivation, anger and rage, overreaction to criticism, feelings of being unable to satisfy ideals, poor self-esteem or guilt, indecision, lack of concentration or forgetfulness, restlessness and agitation, changes in eating or sleeping patterns, substance abuse, problems with authority, or suicidal thoughts.

Identifying feelings of hopelessness or "meaninglessness" is an important factor in understanding completed and attempted suicide in older children and adolescents (Riesch et al., 2008). Reporting feelings of hopelessness has been found to be an even stronger predictor of suicidal behavior than depression (Donaldson, Spirito, & Farnett, 2000), and may be the strongest predictor of future suicide completions (Fritsch, Donaldson, Spirito, & Plummer, 2000).

Social Relationships and Family Influences   The psychosocial characteristics of suicidal ideation are easily recognized by school counselors. Danger signs for higher rates of suicidal ideation are: low self-concept, limited or no supportive friends, isolation from peers, peer conflict, and boyfriend/girlfriend breakup (Prinstein et al., 2000). Adolescent adjustment is also an important component of healthy peer functioning. Adolescents require positive friendships that do not have negative influences such as drug use, criminal activity and juvenile delinquency, or getting in trouble at school (Galassi & Akos, 2007; Moskos, Halbern, Alder, Kim, & Gray, 2007). Although close friendships can be protective factors in preventing suicidal ideation, it is important to recognize that when deviant behavior is present the close friendship may no longer be preventative but may become a risk factor (Prinstein et al.). Because weak peer relationships are an important forecaster of suicidal ideations, a school counselor's observational skills are crucial to the process of prevention and intervention (Leslie et al, 2002; Riesch et al., 2008).

Family dysfunctionality is another factor linked with an increase in suicidal ideations. For instance, children who were raised in families with low social support and poor problem solving may show signs of suicidal ideation (Esposito & Clum, 2003; Riesch et al. 2008). Adolescents who do not see themselves as part of the family unit and have more conflicts within the family are also at a greater risk of suicide (Leslie et al., 2002). Other family variables contributing to suicidal ideation are discord between the child and a parent, the death of a close relative, the absence of the father from the home, not residing with a parent, and financial problems within the family (Spirito, Valeri, Boergers, & Donaldson, 2003). Exposure to a relative's suicide can make some adolescents vulnerable to imitating the behavior. A high percentage of those who complete suicide have had a first- or second-degree relative who attempted or completed suicide (Kaczmarek, Hagan, & Kettler, 2006).

Negative early attachment experiences have been indirectly connected to suicidal ideation as well (Bostik & Everall, 2007). Lack of attachment can have adverse effects on self-esteem, affect-regulation, relationship functioning, and expectations for the future. However, early childhood attachments can also protect the adolescent from suicidal ideation (DiFilippo & Overholser, 2000). As mandated reporters of child abuse, it is important for school counselors to be aware that abuse within the family can be a risk factor for those adolescents who attempt or complete suicide (Moskos, Olson, Halbern, Keller, & Gray, 2005).

Substance Abuse   When drug use goes beyond experimentation, it can have serious health consequences that may lead to suicidal ideation. For instance, adolescent substance abuse (see chapter 5) and suicidal ideation (Riesch et al, 2008) are positively correlated, just as the combination of substance abuse and depression tends to elevate the threat of suicide (Prinstein et al., 2000; Spirito et al., 2003). Other risk factors such as antisocial behavior, aggressive behavior, and affective disorders, when combined with substance abuse, are extremely dangerous, frequently leading to suicidal ideation (American Foundation for Suicide Prevention, 2009b; Csorba et al., 2003; Kaczmarek et al., 2006). While boys are more likely to use solvents, the drugs of choice for girls experiencing suicidal ideation are alcohol or cocaine (as "crack" or in other forms) (Leslie et al., 2002).

Finally, substance abuse coupled with depression and conduct disorders may lead to low academic achievement and failure at school. Being aware of each student's truancy problems and low grade point averages are important ways in which counselors can help identify those students who are at risk for substance abuse and potential suicidal ideation (Hallfors, Cho, Brodish, Flewelling, & Khatapoush, 2006).

Stress   Students who experience high levels of stress have a greater likelihood of experiencing suicidal ideation (Riesch et al., 2008). The stresses of adolescent life may include such stressors as identity and sexuality confusion, and the desire to run away (Leslie et al., 2002; Moskos et al., 2005). It is not uncommon for runaway youth to experience suicidal ideation, and some attempt suicide. Female runaways are more likely to attempt suicide and have a greater number of suicide attempts over their lifetime. Sadly, these youth often lack social and family support, experience abuse and loneliness, and may suffer from mood disorders. As school counselors assess whether students are at risk for suicidal ideation, these factors need to be considered (Leslie et al.; Savin-Williams & Ream, 2003).

Sexual Identity   Gay and bisexual youth are at a higher risk of attempting suicide than their straight peers (Silenzio, Pena, Duberstein, Cerel, & Knox, 2007). It is estimated they are 20 to 42 percent more likely to attempt suicide. Gay and bisexual youth often have less social and familial support, are at a higher risk of negative health behaviors, and are more likely to have been victimized, threatened, and alienated by their families (e.g., forced out of the family home). Rather than their own choices leading to suicidal ideation, it is others' negative reactions to homosexual preferences that may put gay and lesbian youth at higher risk for suicidality (Leslie et al., 2002; Savin-Williams & Ream, 2003).

Professional school counselors might consider the social disintegration model when conceptualizing childhood and youth suicide (Riesch et al., 2008). Students are more likely to have suicidal ideations when they demonstrate ongoing problems in five areas: intrapersonal (e.g., poor ways of coping with problems), interpersonal (weak family communication, functioning and caring), peer networks (lack of school connectedness and climate, educational aspirations, ease of developing friends), physicality (physical development, gender, and ethnicity issues), and participation in risky behaviors (substance use, weapons).

RECOMMENDATIONS FOR SCHOOL
COUNSELING PRACTICE

What can school counselors do to prevent and intervene if students exhibit these warning signs? Professional school counselors need practical, research-based suggestions on how to carefully and effectively prevent suicides and intervene with students who experience suicidal ideations. Of course, before any school counseling assistance is provided to students and their families, the legal and ethical issues must be considered (see Capuzzi, 2002, for a detailed discussion).

Prevention

In 2001, United States Surgeon General David Satcher (2001) brought to light the dire need for mental health services for children and youth. Satcher referred to this lack as "a national health crisis" and called upon agencies, including schools, to provide effective prevention services. A survey asking adolescents about mental health interventions found that teens see themselves as needing intervention, but they did not know where to find and access mental health services (Kirchner, Yoder, Kramer, Lindsey, & Thrush, 2000; Zimmer-Gembeck, Alexander, & Nystrom, 1997). As every child is mandated to attend school, it seems natural that schools are the first line of defense against childhood mental illness, including depression and suicide (Doll & Cummings, 2008; Reis & Cornell, 2008).

Traditionally, suicide prevention activities tend to be implemented in schools after an attempted or completed suicide brings the issue to the crisis stage (Butler, 1994). These prevention programs are not likely to be effective, and in fact may create more stress than they alleviate. Authoritative health care organizations recommend that suicide prevention programs, in order to be successful, should take in to account the mental health of all children and adolescents, not just those perceived to be at-risk (e.g., Center for Disease Control and Prevention, 2009; World Health Organization (2000). A good place to begin is with the "Suicide Prevention Basics" available online from the Suicide Prevention Resource Center (2005).

When discussing suicide prevention in schools, school counselors should note who in the school community can help with prevention activities. Because classroom teachers are in regular contact with students, school counselors and teachers together are responsible for the prevention of suicide. Adopting a school-wide educational approach is beneficial. For example, school counselors and other educators need to be aware of the issues faced by different student groups and know what information to disseminate when coordinating prevention strategies. Certain educators may feel anxious about discussing students' feelings with them, especially when those feelings might lead to suicidal thoughts (Holman, 1997). Research shows that talking about suicide does not encourage the act (Gould et al., 2005; Holman, 1997; Mann et al., 2005), nor does screening for suicidality create or encourage suicidal ideation or behavior (Mann et al.).

With school counselors' large case loads, it is crucial that other educators, especially teachers and administrators, be trained to identify and deal with depression and suicide ideology (Reis & Cornell, 2008). Despite the fact that teachers are on the front line, teacher and administrator preparation programs generally do not offer extensive guidance on how to identify the warning signs of depression and suicide (King, Price, Telljohann, & Wahl, 1999; World Health Organization (2000). When teachers are knowledgeable about these signs and related community resources, form strong relationships with their students, and collaborate closely with school counselors, they become a safeguard against student self-harm (Kirchner, et al., 2000). Educators can attend in-services on to handle difficult emotional situations and help troubled students to feel less stigmatized when seeking help from adults (Mann et al., 2005).

Moreover, as developmentally appropriate, professional school counselors can readily team up with teachers to address preventive health topics (e.g., drug and alcohol use, home and school violence, value of exercise and nutrition, and sexually transmitted diseases) that may have an indirect effect on suicidal ideations (Adams, Husting, Zahnd, & Ozer, 2009). Students should be made aware of the risks of suicide and the resources available to them and know where to turn when a friend confides in them about having suicidal thoughts. Above all, training for students, teachers, and parents needs to take place before a crisis occurs (Moskos et al., 2005; Reis & Cornell).

Teacher in-services should focus on topics such as an overview of depression, the characteristics and warning signs of child and adolescent depression and suicidality, five common myths about adolescent suicide, responding to a crisis or statement about suicide, and the role of the school counselor in mental health situations (Kirchner et al., 2000; Reis & Cornell, 2008). It is good for teachers to know that when they have concerns about a student, they can refer the student to the counseling office for further support and evaluation. Armed with information and aware that they have the support of other educators and school counselors, teachers are more likely to be proactive in keeping an eye out for students who may require mental health services (Capuzzi, 2002; Reis & Cornell). There are structured prevention training courses available to school counselors and teachers (e.g., QPR Institute at http://www.qprinstitute.com/). Proper training for teachers is vital to identifying students' at-risk behaviors and knowing how that behavior might be associated to depression and suicide. In addition, school administrators can support the process, as they often have information about current family dynamics that may result in a student's suicide attempt.

Educating parents and caregivers is also necessary. Parents need to be aware that when their child or their child's friend mentions suicide, it should not be taken lightly. They should know the warning signs and characteristics of those at risk for suicide. It is also important that parents know what resources are available to them, including, but not limited to, the school counselor (Moskos et al., 2005). A presentation at a Parent Teacher Association meeting might be a useful way to share information and answer questions from families.

In prevention work, the role of the school counselor takes on several dimensions. The school counselor should be involved in all aspects of the prevention, identification, and intervention process in the school. First, counselors must help school administrators understand the need for a crisis plan and for student, teacher, and family education, as well as for prevention and intervention services. Without administrative support and a crisis plan in place, school personnel are largely ineffective. Second, school counselors should lead in-service training for teachers and other educators so they become comfortable identifying the signs of depression and suicidal thoughts and attempts in students. It is essential for counselors to work closely with teachers to recognize students who may be having trouble at home or in school, and make themselves accessible to teachers, administrators, parents, caregivers, and students who may have concerns about themselves or a peer.

Suicide Risk Assessment

Once students arrive at the counseling office, whether the student self-referred or was sent in by an educator, parent/caregiver, or peer/friend, it is time to put the crisis plan into effect. First, the counselor should assess the student. The following are recommendations on how to conduct such a risk appraisal.

When appraising suicidal ideation in students, professional school counselors can use many informative techniques and instruments (see Berman, Jobes, &

Sliverman, 2005; Merrill, 2008, for summaries and reviews). Of course when using these assessment measures, school counselors must be very cautious and work within their scope of practice and training. Although many well-validated and researched instruments are available, many are not appropriate for students under 17 years of age. Additionally, when assessing for risk of suicide, quality consultation is paramount. No counselor should make decisions alone, and even though assessment instruments are helpful in evaluating situations and students, instruments alone are no match for the clinical experience and judgment of the counselor's professional colleagues.

There are some appraisal tools that the counselor/clinician completes and others that require the student (or significant other or family member/peer) to self-report. Whether students are handed a questionnaire to fill out themselves or counselors ask the questions, research has shown that there is little difference between the two approaches in the answers that are given (Kaplan, Asnis, Sanderson, Keswani, DeLecuona, & Joseph, 1994). The major difference found was in current suicidal ideation. Many people felt more comfortable reporting any current thought of suicide on the self-report form. If a student were to verbally answer "no" to current suicidal ideation, it would be best for the school counselor to follow up with either a self-report form or to follow their clinical judgment and contact the appropriate persons as necessary.

There are several instruments counselors can use to assess suicide risk in students. Clinician-completed instruments are designed to assess suicidal ideation in clinical populations. They are scored and interpreted only by highly trained mental health clinicians. Self-report measures can be in the form of paper-and-pencil or computer-based questionnaires, where students, if appropriate, complete the instrument with school counselor assistance and follow-up.

The following are two published examples of widely used, youth-appropriate suicide assessment instruments. Many of the published and unpublished measures are reviewed at the Web site EndingSuicide.com.

- The Suicide Probability Scale (SPS; Cull & Gill, 1982) is a 36-item self-report questionnaire that can be administered to children and youth 13 years and older. Measuring a student's sense of hopelessness, hostility, and suicidal ideation, the SPS uses a 4-point Likert scale and takes approximately 5–10 minutes to complete.

- The Suicidal Ideation Questionnaire (SIQ: Reynolds, 1988) has two versions for youth (SIQ JR for grades 7 through 9 and SIQ for grades 10 through12). The screening instrument takes approximately 5–10 minutes for students to complete.

- There are several unpublished and informal scripted interviews school counselors can use to assess suicide risk (e.g., Adolescent Suicide Interview, Child Suicide Potential Scale, and the Suicidal Behavioral Inventory). Please see the end of this chapter for additional information and resources.

Interviewing students for suicidal ideation is a challenging process and requires extensive training (Merrill, 2008). Because of their knowledge base, professional school counselors connecting with the school psychologist to develop an interview protocol/process is good practice (Debski, Spadafore, Jacob, Poole, & Hixson, 2007). When assessing a student, death needs to be discussed in forthright manner. Counselors must ask difficult questions in a calm, non-judgmental way. They must take seriously every statement students make about attempting or wanting to attempt suicide. Generally, suicide assessment interviews cover these areas: thinking about suicide, making a suicide plan, the means and preparation for a suicide attempt, and the intended place or setting (Merrill). Here are some sample questions a school counselor can ask:

- Are you planning on killing yourself? (This direct question confirms suicidal ideation.)

- Do you have a plan? (Determines how thought-out the suicidal ideation is. If a student does not have a plan, he or she may be seeking help without planning his or her death.)

- Do you have access to the means (e.g., weapons, medications, poisons) to carry out your plan? (This question helps determine the student's access to the means of completion of ideation. For example, students who want to shoot themselves but do not have a gun in the house are less at-risk than students who indicate they are going to shoot themselves and have access to firearms.)

- How long have you been thinking about killing yourself? (With this question the counselor can determine the student's feeling of hopelessness. Students who have been planning their death for a long time generally have difficulty seeing other ways of coping. The longer the suicidal ideation has been there, the more lethal the thoughts can become.)

- Have you tried to kill yourself before? (Students who have made previous attempts are at higher risk.)

- What is going on in your life that would make you choose to end it? (Using open-ended questions allows the student to share some of the issues precipitating suicidal ideation.)

- What are some other ways to deal with this situation besides killing yourself? (This is a way of assessing the student's coping skills and feelings of hopelessness. If a student can see alternatives, this is a good sign.)

- If you did cut your wrists (or swallow poison, or overdose on medication; however the student said he or she would kill himself or herself), who would find you like that? (Again, this question is asking for explicit information about how, where, and when students would kill themselves.)

In short, the above-mentioned questions give the school counselor important information as to the lethality of the suicidal ideation.

Calling attention to details about death and the survivors may make the act more real. The answer to the question also determines the student's state of mind. An answer of "no one" or "a stranger" provides insight into the family dynamics. "I don't know" may indicate that the student may not have thought that far into the dying process. Answers naming parents, a relative, or a family friend should be followed up on by asking, "How would they feel?" This follow-up question hopefully will allow the student to empathize with survivors (Holman, 1997).

Interventions

School counselors also need to support a student's parents and caregivers and perhaps even their siblings. Regardless of the lethality of the suicidal ideation, not only should school administrators be notified, but school counselors should also contact the student's family and involve them in the intervention process (Cohn, 2006). The goal is take immediate protective action (Merrill, 2008).

Parents (including caregivers and guardians) should be told of their student's ideation, including potential lethality. Professional school counselors should ask parents about any access to the means stated in the student's suicide plan and encourage parents to admit their child into psychotherapy, providing referrals as necessary. In addition, parents need to be reminded to take the suicidal ideation seriously and to be empathic when discussing the issue with their child. Parents also need to be given phone numbers to call in the event of a crisis. However, school counselors also need to be aware that providing parents and students with a crisis call center number is not sufficient. If an emergency occurs outside of school hours, they need to immediately go to the local emergency room for care. Crisis call lines are considered a secondary level of care once the school counselor or another mental health professional is involved. That said, parents and students should be encouraged to use the crisis call center via phone or Internet when necessary.

Clinical- vs. School-Based Interventions   Research on effective interventions for suicidal individuals is difficult to conduct well and frequently laden with methodological and ethical concerns (Fristad & Shaver, 2001; Spirito, Stanton, Donaldson, & Boegers, 2002). Obviously, as students receive qualified medical and psychiatric treatment, school counselors do not plan and institute any school-based therapy; doing so would be beyond the scope of their training (American School Counselor Association, 2006). Instead, they serve as a school support person and liaison within and among the student's various systems (e.g., psychologist, family, treatment facility, teachers).

External mental health professionals focus on remediation problem-solving and social skill deficits, while long-term goals tend to center on building self-esteem and interpersonal relationship skills (Fristad & Shaver, 2001). If appropriate, school counselors can scaffold these goals fostering student personal-social competence and resiliency (Masten, Herbers, Cutuli, & Lafavor, 2008). Often just connecting regularly with students for supportive and caring dialogue can be a useful part of the healing process.

Intervention often involves psychopharmacology to manage potential coexisting mental illnesses (e.g., serious depression, bipolar disorder, or other mood disorders) and confront hopelessness. A user-friendly overview of these medications can be found at NIMH's Web site (2009a; also see Table 3.2). Psychotherapy as a component of intervention can reframe cognitive distortions, remedy social problems and teach problem-solving skills. There may also be family involvement in the intervention therapies including, for example, parenting education and family therapy (Brent, 1997; Fristad & Shaver, 2001; Juhnke & Shoffner, 1999; Mann et al., 2005; Ryan, 2005).

While two-thirds of adolescents who received medication for depression remain compliant, only one half of suicidal students keep their first therapy appointment and only one third of those attend more than three counseling sessions (Fristad & Shaver, 2001; King et al., 1997). School counselor follow-up is therefore imperative, letting students know that these therapy appointments are important to attend at all times, not just when they are in crisis. Additionally, checking in helps counselors ascertain whether students are treatment-compliant. If not, counselors should contact the parent or caregiver to reinforce with the student that mental health treatment is not optional. If the family is noncompliant and fails to do their part, the counselor must then contact child protective services and report their noncompliance as child endangerment.

Postvention

If prevention and intervention strategies are not successful and a student commits suicide, postvention strategies will need to be employed. As with all stages in dealing with student suicide, a postvention plan should be in place before it is needed (AAS, 1998; Debski, Spadafore, Jacob, Poole, & Hixson, 2007; Maples, Packman, Abney, Daugherty, Casey, & Pirtle, 2005). Numerous approaches are available online and in professional literature (e.g., TEAM; Roberts, Lepkowski, & Davidson, 1998; Mental Health America of Wisconsin's Wisconsin Components of School-Based Suicide Prevention, Intervention, Postvention Model, n.d.). When planning a postvention, several issues must be considered.

The TEAM approach to postvention is a good model to follow (Maples et al., 2005; Roberts et al., 1998). This strategy sets up a team (T) to handle the postvention, where a CAPT Team of counselors (C), administrators (A), parents/caregivers (P), and teachers (T) are involved (Maples et al.). TEAM establishes (E) postvention procedures, including how students and staff will be informed of the suicide who will handle the media and what information will be provided to the media, and what the coordination process between the surviving family members and the school district and its existing policies will be. The organization of any planned memorial services should be addressed by the team. Furthermore, there must be arrangements made (A) for an external support network (i.e., a local crisis team) to be brought into the school. For example, support small groups should be organized up front, making sure the lines of communication are clear, indicating who will facilitate the groups, which students will be invited, and how long the groups will be available. When and how debriefing meetings will be conducted and by whom must also be determined.

There are four indiscrete stages that should be considered while arranging outside support personnel (Brammer, Abrego, & Shostrom, 1993). The first stage is shock and disorganization, when students and staff experience denial and try coping with confusion. During this stage the students need to be made aware, if they were not previously, of the resources provided by the CAPT Team. The second phase includes the opportunity for survivors to express anguish and remorse. In the third stage, students need to have an opportunity to explore the meaning of loss. The fourth stage is marked by the emergence of new goals, specifically, creating new goals for oneself and the group (Brammer et al.). The counseling members of the CAPT Team should address these stages while arranging support. A good way to address these stages of grief and remorse is within small counseling groups.

In order to deal with the confusion that follows a completed suicide, information should not be given in groups larger than a normal class size. The information provided should be consistent and truthful, straightforward but with limited detail (AAS, 1998). The final component in the TEAM postvention approach is the monitoring (M) of progress (i.e., Are other students at risk? How will future prevention and interventions be conducted?). When applied well, the TEAM approach is an effective method for dealing with the aftermath of a suicide.

SUMMARY

There are many challenges in identifying students who are at risk for suicidal ideation and suicide completion. Because the school provides ongoing access to children and adolescents, as seen in the case study of Megan, it is a natural setting for prevention as well as for early identification and intervention (Hallfors et al., 2006). Not only had Megan described herself as feeling disconnected to her parents and feeling isolated from peers, she showed signs of depression, hopelessness, and the inability to control her suicidal thoughts and impulses; above all, she had developed a plan. With knowledge of the warning signs of suicidal ideation and aware of the value of early intervention, Megan's school counselor was able to start a discussion with Megan and her mother, facilitate positive communications between them, and get Megan the appropriate treatment she needed. Megan also received her school counselor's support, participating in a small group for self-esteem issues.

The key for school counselors is to be aware of the characteristics which put students at risk, identify students with suicidal ideation, and know the interventions that can be effective in preventing student suicide. In the event of a completed suicide, an organized plan must be in place to minimize the risk of future suicides in the school population while dealing with the emotional impact on educators and peers of the loss of a classmate. It is important to remember that while there is only one death in a suicide, there are many victims (Parsons, 1996). Professional school counselors influence whether suicidal students and their families and peers can be appropriately handled in the educational environment. In addition to the material presented above and in the chapter references, Table 8.1 provides useful Web sites to support school counselors with students at risk for suicide and their families. With this information and skills at their disposal, school counselors can play a major role in saving their students' lives.

TABLE 8.1   Web Resources for Professional School Counselors

■ American Association for Suicidology	■ http://www.suicidology.org/web/guest/home
■ American Foundation for Suicide Prevention	■ http://www.afsp.org/
■ Comprehensive list of child and adolescent appropriate screening instruments	■ www.endingsuicide.com
■ National Institute of Mental Health	■ http://www.nimh.nih.gov/health/topics/suicide-prevention/index.shtml
■ Suicide Prevention Resource Center	■ http://www.sprc.org/

REFERENCES

Adams, S. H., Husting, S., Zahnd, E., & Ozer, E. M. (2009). Adolescent preventive services: Rates and disparities in preventive health topics covered during routine medical care in a California sample. *Journal of Adolescent Health, 44,* 536–545.

American Association of Suicidology (AAS). (1998, Fall). *New Link, 24,* 3, 126–128.

American Association of Suicidology (AAS). (2008). *Youth suicide fact sheet.* Retrieved June 9, 2009, from http://www.suicidology.org/c/document_library/get_file?folderId=232&name=DLFE-24.pdf

American Foundation for Suicide Prevention. (2009a). *Facts and figures.* Retrieved June 9, 2009, from http://www.afsp.org/index.cfm?fuseaction=home.viewPage&page_id=04EA1254-BD31-1FA3-C549D77E6CA6AA37

American Foundation for Suicide Prevention. (2009b). *Risk factors for suicide.* Retrieved June 9, 2009, from http://www.afsp.org/index.cfm?fuseaction=home.viewPage&page_id=05147440-E24E-E376-BDF4BF8BA6444E76

American Foundation for Suicide Prevention. (2009c). *Warning signs of suicide.* Retrieved June 9, 2009, from http://www.afsp.org/index.cfm?fuseaction=home.viewPage&page_id=0519EC1A-D73A-8D90-7D2E9E2456182D66

American Psychiatric Association. (2000). *Diagnostic and statistical manual of mental disorders—Text revision.* Washington, DC: Author.

American School Counselor Association. (2006). *The ASCA National Model: A framework for school counseling programs.* Retrieved June 10, 2009, from http://www.schoolcounselor.org/files/Natl%20Model%20Exec%20Summary_final.pdf

Berman, A. L., Jobes, D. A., & Sliverman, M. M. (2005). *Adolescent suicide: Assessment and intervention* (2nd ed.). Washington, DC: American Psychological Association.

Bostik, K. E., & Everall, R. D. (2007). Healing from suicide: Adolescent perceptions of attachment relationships. *British Journal of Guidance & Counselling, 35,* 79–96.

Brammer, L. M., Abrego, P., & Shostrom, E. (1993). *Therapeutic counseling and psychotherapy* (6th ed.). Upper Saddle River, NJ: Prentice Hall.

Brent, D. A. (1997). The aftercare of adolescents with deliberate self-harm. *Journal of Child Psychology Psychiatry, 38,* 277–286.

Bridge, J. A., Greenhouse, J. B., & Weldon, A. H. (2008). Suicide trends among youths aged 10 to 19 years in the United States, 1996-2005. *Journal of the American Medical Association (JAMA), 300*, 1025–1026. Retrieved June 9, 2009, from http://jama. ama-assn.org/cgi/reprint/300/9/1025

Caballero, J., & Nahata, M. C. (2005). Selective serotonin-reuptake inhibitors and suicidal ideation and behavior in children. *American Journal of Health-System Pharmacy, 62*, 864–867.

Capuzzi, D. (2002). Legal and ethical challenges in counseling suicidal students – Special issue: legal and ethical issues in school counseling. *Professional School Counseling, 6*, 36–45.

Center for Disease Control and Prevention (CDC). (2006). *Suicide fact sheet.* Retrieved June 10, 2009, from http://www.cdc.gov/ncipc/pub-res/Suicide%20Fact%20Sheet.pdf

Center for Disease Control and Prevention (CDC). (2009). *Preventing suicide: Program activities guide.* Retrieved June 10, 2009, from http://www.cdc.gov/ViolencePrevention/pub/PreventingSuicide.html

Cohn, A. (2006). Preventing youth suicide: Tips for parents and educators. *NASP Communiqué, 35*(4), n.p. Retrieved June 10, 2009, from http://www.nasponline.org/publications/cq/cq354suicide.aspx

Csorba, J., Rózsa, S., Gádoros, J., Vetró, E. K., Sarungi, E., Makra, J., et al. (2003). Suicidal depressed vs. non-suicidal depressed adolescents: differences in recent psychopathology. *Journal of Affective Disorders, 74*, 229–236.

Cull, J. G., & Gill, W. S. (1982). *Suicide Probability Scale manual.* Los Angeles: Western Psychological Services.

Debski, J., Spadafore, C. D., Jacob, S., Poole, D. A., & Hixson, M. D. (2007). Suicide intervention: Training, roles, and knowledge of school psychologists. *Psychology in the Schools, 44*, 157–170.

Doll, B., & Cummings, J. A. (2008). Why population-based services are essential for school mental health, and how to make them happen in your school. In B. Doll & J. A. Cummings (Eds.), *Transforming school mental health services population-based approaches to promoting the competency and wellness of children* (pp. 1–19). Thousand Oaks, CA: Corwin.

Donaldson, D., Spirito, A., & Farnett, E. (2000). The role of perfectionism and depressive cognitions in understanding the hopelessness experienced by adolescent suicide attempters. *Child Psychiatry and Human Development, 31*, 99–111.

DiFilippo, J. M., & Overholser, J. C. (2000). Suicidal ideation in adolescent psychiatric inpatients as associated with depression and attachment relationships. *Journal of Clinical Child Psychology, 29*, 155–166.

Esposito, C. L., & Clum, G. A. (2003). The relative contribution of diagnostic and psychosocial factors in the prediction of adolescent suicidal ideation. *Journal of Clinical Child and Adolescent Psychology, 32*, 386–395.

Fristad, M.A., & Shaver, A.E. (2001). Psychosocial interventions for suicidal children and adolescents. *Depression and Anxiety, 14*, 192–197.

Fritsch, S., Donaldson, D., Spirito, A., & Plummer, B. (2000). Personality characteristics of adolescent suicide attempters. *Child Psychiatry and Human Development, 30*, 219–235.

Galassi, J. P., & Akos, P. (2007). *Strengths-based school counseling*. Mahweh, NJ: Lawrence Erlbaum.

Gould, M. S., Marrocco, F. A., Kleinman, M., Thomas, J. G., Mostkoff, K., Cote, J., et al. (2005). Evaluating iatrogenic risk of youth suicide screening programs. *Journal of the American Medical Association, 293*, 1635–1643.

Hallfors, D., Cho, H., Brodish, P. H., Flewelling, R., & Khatapoush, S. (2006). Identifying high school students "at risk" for substance use and other behavioral problems: Implications for prevention. *Substance Use & Misuse, 41*, 1–15.

Holman, W. D. (1997). "Who would find you?" A question for working with suicidal children and adolescents. *Children and Adolescent Social Work Journal, 14*, 129–137.

Hull, D. (2009). *School counselors, psychologists play critical role*. Retrieved June 10, 2009, from http://www.mercurynews.com/localnewsheadlines/ci_12556018

Juhnke, G. A., & Shoffner, M. F. (1999). The family debriefing model: An adapted critical incident stress debriefing for parents and older sibling suicide survivors. *The Family Journal: Counseling and Therapy for Couples and Families, 7*, 342–348.

Kaplan, M. L., Asnis, G. M., Sanderson, W.C., Keswani, L., DeLecuona, J. M., & Joseph, S. (1994). Suicide assessment: Clinical interview versus self-report. *Journal of Clinical Psychology, 50*, 294–298.

Kaczmarek, T. L., Hagan, M. P., & Kettler, R. J. (2006). Screening for suicide among juvenile delinquents: Reliability and validity evidence for the suicide screening inventory (SSI). *International Journal of Offender Therapy and Comparative Criminology, 50*, 204–217.

King, K. A., Price, J. H., Telljohann, S. K., & Wahl, J. (1999). High school health teachers perceived self-efficacy in identifying students at risk for suicide, *Journal of School Health, 69*, 202–207.

Kirchner, J. E., Yoder, M. K., Kramer, T. L., Lindsey, M. S., & Thrush, C. R. (2000). Development of an educational program to increase school personnel's awareness about child and adolescent depression, *Education, 121*, 235–247.

Leslie, M. B., Stein, J. A., & Rotheram-Borus, M. J. (2002). Sex-specific predictors of suicidality among runaway youth. *Journal of Clinical Child and Adolescent Psychology, 31*, 27–40.

Mann, J. J., Apter, A., Bertolote, J., Beautrais, A., Currier, D., Haas, A., et al. (2005). Suicidal prevention strategies: A systematic review. *Journal of the American Medical Association, 294*, 2064–2074.

Maples, M. F., Packman, J., Abney, P., Daugherty, R. F., Casey, J. A., & Pirtle, L. (2005). Suicide by teenagers in middle school: A postvention team approach. *Journal of Counseling & Development, 83*, 397–405.

Masten, A. S., Herbers, J. E., Cutuli, J. J., & Lafavor, T. L. (2008). Promoting competence and resilience in the school context. *Professional School Counseling, 12*, 76–84.

McIntosh, J. L. (2009). *USA state suicide rates and rankings among the elderly and young*, 2006. Retrieved June 9, 2009, from http://www.suicidology.org/c/document_library/get_file?folderId=228&name=DLFE-144.pdf

Mental Health America of Wisconsin. (n.d.). *The Wisconsin components of school-based suicide Prevention, Intervention, postvention model*. Retrieved June 10, 2009, from http://www.mhawisconsin.org/Uploads/spschoolbased/iiicomponentsofsbspostv.doc

Merrill, K. M. (2008). *Behavioral, social, and emotional assessment of children and adolescents* (3rd ed.). New York: Lawrence Erlbaum.

Moskos, M. A., Halbern, S. R., Alder, S., Kim, H., & Gray, D. (2007). Utah youth suicide study: Evidence-based suicide prevention for juvenile offenders. *Journal of Law & Family Studies, 10*, 127–145.

Moskos, M. A., Olson, L., Halbern, S, Keller, T., & Gray, D. (2005). Utah youth suicide study: Psychological autopsy. *Suicide and Life-Threatening Behavior, 35*, 536–546.

National Center for Injury Prevention and Control. (2008). *Suicide prevention.* Retrieved June 9, 2009, from http://www.cdc.gov/ncipc/dvp/suicide/youthsuicide.htm

National Institute of Mental Health (NIMH). (2009a). *Medications.* Retrieved June 10, 2009, from http://www.nimh.nih.gov/health/publications/medications/complete-index.shtml

National Institute of Mental Health (NIMH). (2009b). *Suicide in the US: Statistics and prevention* (Report from 2004). Retrieved June 8, 2009, from http://www.nimh.nih.gov/health/publications/suicide-in-the-us-statistics-and-prevention/index.shtml

National Mental Health Information Center. (2006). *Mood disorders.* Retrieved June 9, 2009, from http://mentalhealth.samhsa.gov/publications/allpubs/ken98-0049/default.asp

Olfson, M., Shaffer, D, Marcus, S., & Greenberg, T. (2003). Relationship between antidepressant medication treatment and suicide in adolescents. *Archives of General Psychiatry, 60*, 978–982.

Parsons, R. (1996). Student suicide: The counselor's postvention role. *Elementary School Guidance and Counseling, 31*, 77–80.

Prinstein, M. J., Boergers, J., Spirito, A., Little, T. D., & Grapentine, W. L. (2000). Peer functioning, family dysfunction, and psychological symptoms in a risk factor model for adolescent inpatients' suicidal ideation severity. *Journal of Clinical Child Psychology, 29*, 392–405.

Reynolds, W. (1988). *Suicidal Ideation Questionnaire: Professional manual.* Odessa, FL: Psychological Assessment Resources.

Reis, C., & Cornell, D. (2008). An evaluation of suicide gatekeeper training for school counselors and teachers. *Professional School Counseling, 11*, 386–394.

Riesch, S. K., Jacobson, G. Sawdey, L., Anderson, J., & Henriques, J. (2008). Suicide ideation among later elementary school-aged youth. *Journal of Psychiatric & Mental Health Nursing, 15*, 263–277.

Roberts, R., Lepkowski, W., & Davidson, K. (1998). Dealing with the aftermath of a student suicide: A T.E.A.M approach. *NAASP Bulletin, 82*, 53–59.

Ryan, N. D. (2005). Treatment of depression in children and adolescents. *Lancet, 366*, 933–940.

Satcher, D. (2001). *Report of the Surgeon General's Conference on Children's Mental Health: A national action agenda for children's mental health.* Retrieved June 10, 2009, from http://www.surgeongeneral.gov/topics/cmh/childreport.htm

Savin-Williams, R. C., & Ream, G. L. (2003). Suicide attempts among sexual-minority male youth. *Journal of Clinical Child and Adolescent Psychology, 32*, 509–522.

Silenzio, V. M. B., Pena, J. B., Duberstein, P. R., Cerel, J., & Knox, K. L. (2007). Sexual orientation and risk factors for suicidal ideation and suicide attempts among adolescents and young adults. *American Journal of Public Health, 97*, 2017–2019.

Spirito, A., Stanton, C., Donaldson, D., & Boergers, J. (2002). Treatment-as-usual for adolescent suicide attempters: Implications for the choice of comparison groups in psychotherapy research. *Journal of Clinical Child and Adolescent Psychology, 31,* 41–47.

Spirito, A., Valeri, S., Boergers, J., & Donaldson, D. (2003). Predictors of continued suicidal behavior in adolescents following a suicide attempt. *Journal of Clinical Child and Adolescent Psychology, 32,* 284–289.

Suicide Prevention Resource Center. (2005). *Suicide prevention basics.* Retrieved June 10, 2009, from http://www.sprc.org/suicide_prev_basics/index.asp

World Health Organization. (2000). *Preventing suicide: A resource for teachers and other school staff.* Retrieved June 10, 2009, from http://www.who.int/mental_health/media/en/62.pdf

Zimmer-Gembeck, M. J., Alexander, T., & Nystrom, R. J. (1997). Adolescents report their need for and use of health care services. *Journal of Adolescent Health, 21,* 388–399.

Chapter 9

Learning Disabilities

GLENN W. LAMBIE, KARA P. IEVA,
STACY VAN HORN, JONATHAN H. OHRT,
SALLY LEWIS, AND B. GRANT HAYES

University of Central Florida

S tudents with learning disabilities often experience many challenges that may increase their chances for impaired academic, vocational, and social-emotional development. In collaboration with other educators, professional school counselors can provide comprehensive counseling services to students diagnosed with various types of learning disabilities. However, they may not do this at all well. Romano (2006) found that a majority of school counselors from certain parts of the United States had minimal or no education on how to assist students with learning disabilities on 504 plans. Counselors reported feeling ill-equipped to address educational activities that could support classroom learning or serve as a consultant to the school staff on learning disability issues. It is probably a safe assumption that most professional school counselors across the country have similar perceptions of their skill set at some time or another.

This chapter is intended to assist in filling this knowledge gap. The chapter starts off with two real-world student case studies. Then it summarizes the characteristics of learning disabilities, including terminology and definitional issues, prognosis, and observable warning signs. Subsequently, the legal issues applicable to learning-disabilities education are reviewed. In the final section, collaborative school-based intervention strategies are presented and discussed.

Stacy: An Elementary School-Based Case Study

Stacy was referred to the school counselor by her first grade teacher. The teacher described Stacy as having difficulty associating sounds with letters. Stacy started the year exceedingly motivated and eager to learn to read, but was experiencing great difficulty. The teacher also explained that she had spoken with Stacy's parents, Martha and Gary, and they too indicated that they were noticing difficulties when they practiced reading with Stacy before her bedtime. Recently, Stacy has become withdrawn in class and unwilling to complete her work. The teacher additionally noted that last week's lesson was learning to tell time, and when Stacy became frustrated with the concept, she turned over the clock she was using and refused to participate, which was out of character for her.

As a result of the meeting with Stacy's teacher, the school counselor decided to take two steps toward action. Her first step was to invite Stacy to her office to talk and to introduce herself. During that meeting, Stacy expressed how she often felt upset with school. Stacy indicated that school used to be "something I really liked," but had since turned into something "I don't want to do any more, but I like my teacher." The counselor concluded their meeting by explaining to Stacy that the next step was for her was to call Stacy's parents and schedule a Child Study Team (CST) meeting. The counselor then called Stacy's parents to express her concerns and to describe the CST meeting and invite Stacy's parents to attend. She also provided Stacy's parents with resources related to educational disabilities and contacted all of Stacy's teachers, the school's "exceptional education" coordinator, the school psychologist, and the school's social worker regarding the meeting.

Marcus: A High-School-Based Case Study

Marcus is a tenth-grade student referred to the school counselor by his geometry teacher. The teacher indicated that Marcus was generally an average student but had become withdrawn, no longer participating in cooperative learning activities. She had recently attended an Individual Education Program (IEP) Team meeting in which Marcus had been placed into Resource Science and History classes. She wondered if this change in his class placement had anything to do with his change in her classroom. She also indicated that Marcus shook and did a lot of tapping on the desk surface when taking quizzes and tests, and felt that maybe he needed to talk with someone.

The following day, the counselor met with Marcus. He explained to Marcus that his IEP was intended to support his academic achievement, but that as his counselor, he was there to discuss any issues that may be going on in Marcus's life. At the initial meeting, the counselor was able to establish a level of rapport with Marcus and discuss some of his interests and dislikes. Marcus explained that he loved music and band, but since his IEP mandated he take a double block of reading classes, he was unable to fit band into his schedule. The counselor spoke with the band director to see if it was possible for Marcus to come to the after school band practices, since it did not fit in to his class schedule. The band director agreed, arranging for Marcus to meet with him later that day to discuss his addition to the band.

Two weeks later, Marcus came back to the counselor's office to check in and talk. At this time, Marcus was able to share that he did not like participating in his classes because he was embarrassed and did not want his peers to know he had a learning disability and had problems reading.

CHARACTERISTICS OF LEARNING DISABILITIES

Even after looking at these case studies and their own real-world experiences, school counselors are often unclear as to what actually constitutes a learning disability and what a learning disability might look like in schools.

Defining Learning Disabilities

For the purposes of this chapter, we are focusing on specific learning disabilities (LDs). Although this definition has come under scrutiny of late (Kavale, Spaulding, & Beam, 2009), the Learning Disabilities Association of America (LDA; 2004a) continues to define a learning disability as a "neurologically-based processing problem. These processing problems can interfere with learning basic skills such as reading, writing, or math calculating, or interfere with higher level skills such as organization, time planning, and abstract reasoning" (p.1). The Council for Exceptional Children (CEC; 2007a) stated that "weaker academic achievement, particularly in reading, written language, and math, is perhaps the most fundamental characteristic of LD. Significant deficits often exist in memory, metacognition, and social skills as well" (p. 1).

The National Information Center for Children and Youth with Disabilities (NICHCY, 2004) noted that there are specific types of processing problems relating to LDs that are identified by processing dysfunctions, including (a) input, (b) integration or organization, (c) memory, and (d) output. Input processing relates to information processing carried to the brain by means of the senses, such as the eyes (visual perception) and ears (auditory perception). After information has been input into the brain, three tasks must be carried out in order for a person to make sense of the information (integrate or organize it). Integration or organization processing involves three stages, including sequencing (processing in appropriate order), abstraction (inferring meaning from the information), and organization (assimilating and accommodating information into the current scheme). Memory processing relates to a person's ability to retain information and may be categorized as working memory, short-term memory, and long-term memory. Output processing relates to an individual's ability to communicate both orally (language disabilities) and using muscle activity (motor disabilities; LDA, 2004a; National Dissemination Center for Children with Disabilities, 2009). LDs do not include processing problems primarily caused by visual, hearing, or motor disabilities. However, students with such exceptional education diagnoses may also have LDs.

Prevalence

There is some debate about the prevalence rates of LD in the United States (Goldstein & Schwebach, 2009), but some data are relatively solid. For example, an estimated 51% of children identified with special needs have an LD (McEachern, 2004). Additionally, the CEC (2007a) noted that students with LDs in the United States who are receiving services in exceptional education have more than doubled in the past 30 years. LDs are common, with an estimated 4% to 6% of public school students being identified with the diagnosis of an LD (LDA, 2004b). However, NICHCY (2004) noted that "as many as 1 out of every 5 people in the United States has a learning disability" (p. 2). The U.S. Department of Education (2006) concluded that the percentage of students receiving exceptional education and related services for LDs (the largest disability category) was 5.59%. A slightly higher LD prevalence rate across the 50 states (mean state prevalence = 5.76%, standard deviation = 1.19) was reported by National Research Center on Learning Disabilities (2007). Some experts in the education field speculate that for children between the ages of 6 and 17, 5% to 10% of children will be diagnosed with an LD (CEC, 2007a). Due to the prevalence of the diagnosis of LDs, it is imperative for professional school counselors to be knowledgeable about this category of disability and its potential impact on a student's academic achievement and social-emotional development.

Prognosis

The potential for poor academic, career, and social-emotional development increases with the diagnosis of an LD (Rock & Leff, 2007). Students with a diagnosed learning disability tend to have a lower school completion rate than general education students (Kortering & Christenson, 2009). Additionally, NICHCY (2004) noted that an LD is a lifelong condition that may require special understanding and assistance throughout grade school and high school and beyond. Putnam (2007) suggested that students with LDs are at greater risk for social maladjustment and involvement in risk-taking behaviors (e.g., suicide, substance abuse, sexual activity) than their non-disabled peers. Shechtman and Katz (2007) noted that students with an LD often have poorly defined self-concepts, low self-esteem, higher levels of loneliness and depression, and an increased propensity to be involved in gangs, legal infractions, and substance abuse (Vernon, 2009). By definition, LDs tend to have a significant impact on a student's holistic life outside of the classroom, interfering not only with academic work but also with students' games, daily activities, and friendships (LDA, 2004b). Horowitz (2005) concluded that students with LDs struggle with understanding and managing their own emotions. The potential impact of the diagnosis of an LD on a student's social-emotional development may contribute to low levels of motivation that often lead to having lower career and educational aspiration compared to peers (Kaffenberger & Seligman, 2007). Therefore, students with an LD need support services from their school counselors to promote holistic development and achievement.

Observable Warning Signs—Internalizing
and Externalizing Behaviors

In addition to struggling academically, students with LDs often exhibit problematic behaviors. Teachers, parents and caregivers, and the school counselor can often become frustrated or confused as to why a student is not succeeding.

Teachers sometimes view students with LDs as unmotivated or less competent than their peers (Meltzer, Katzir-Cohen, Miller, & Roditi, 2001). Additionally, teachers may not believe that students with LDs are putting forth a sufficient amount of effort. Often teachers, parents and caregivers, and school counselors have misconceptions about a student's behaviors; therefore, it is important for counselors to be aware of the potential signs and behaviors exhibited by students with potential undiagnosed LDs.

Students with LDs often express feelings of frustration or a lack of control (Rodis, 2001). These feelings may lead to disruptive or immature behavior (e.g., being "bossy") or lack of self-control (Steedly, Schwartz, Levin, & Luke, 2008). Students with LDs may also experience difficulty interpreting social cues and others' moods or feelings, leading them to make comments inappropriate to the time or place (National Center for Learning Disabilities [NCLD], 2006).

Students with LDs often have difficulty in social situations, especially when faced with embarrassment, group pressure, and unexpected challenges. Furthermore, they may have difficulty expressing their feelings and emotions and may have difficulty communicating in general (e.g., they can become consumed by details in a conversation and cannot "get to the point"; NCLD). Finally, students with LDs often exhibit poor impulse control and engage in risk-taking behaviors significantly more often than their non-disabled peers (Putnam, 2007). Therefore, some behavioral problems that school counselors and other educators observe may indirectly contribute to a student's learning disability.

A disability label can often result in students feeling different or isolated from their peers (Witherell & Rodis, 2001). Students with LDs are frequently the victims of bullying (Heinrichs, 2003) and report feeling isolated and anxious in class and disrespected by teachers (Medina & Luna, 2004). Consequently, students with LDs often experience negative feelings about themselves (e.g., shame, anger, and low self-esteem), poor self-concept, depression, and difficulty with interpersonal relationships and in social situations (Shechtman & Katz, 2007; Shechtman & Pastor, 2005). Students with learning disabilities may be doubtful of their own abilities (i.e., they may attribute their successes to outside influences or luck rather than hard work). Students with LDs may also have trouble evaluating their personal-social challenges and strengths (NCLD, 2006).

Social skills deficits, including the failure to establish and maintain friendships and the inability to interpret social cues, may contribute to a student with learning disabilities developing a negative self-image (Horowitz, 2005). Students who are teased or bullied by peers due to a lack of understanding about learning differences can also contribute to low self-esteem. The social-emotional effects of learning disabilities are unique to the individual. In general, though, students with LDs often feel dissatisfaction at school and have an increased likelihood of dropping out (Kaffenberger & Seligman, 2007). These students are often depressed and anxious due to the challenges associated with their disability. Both the externalizing and internalizing behaviors identified in the research are areas the school counselor must be aware of, and be prepared to support students with LDs. For more extensive technical information about the characteristics of learning disabilities, readers are encouraged to review Goldstein and Schwebach (2009).

LEGAL ISSUES AND LEGISLATION GOVERNING LEARNING DISABILITIES

To address the needs of persons with learning disabilities, the government has repeatedly enacted legislation at the federal level. These laws include Section 504 of the Rehabilitation Act of 1973, the Americans with Disabilities Act of 1990 (ADA), and the Individuals with Disabilities Education Improvement Act (IDEIA [2004]; PL 108–146), formerly known as the Education of All Handicapped Children Act of 1975 (PL 94–142, 20 U.S.C Section 1400 [d]). According to Schmidt (2008), the two federal statutes that have had the most impact on school counselors are Section 504 and IDEIA. Additionally, Lambie and Williamson (2004) noted that federal civil rights laws (Section 504 and ADA) and exceptional education legislation (IDEIA [PL 108–146]) expanded the role of professional school counselors in exceptional education, including collaboration in appropriate placement services and IEPs, and providing counseling and consultation services to students diagnosed with exceptionalities and their families. Table 9.1 includes exceptional education terms, acronyms, and brief definitions to assist school counselors in understanding the language of exceptional education.

Civil Rights Legislation

Two federal civil rights laws (Section 504 [1973] and ADA [1990]) significantly relate to the services schools and school counselors are able to provide to students with LDs. Valente and Valente (2001) suggest that Section 504 and ADA "are essentially negative prohibitions against disability-based discrimination" (p. 246). The following section provides a brief introduction to Section 504 and ADA for professional school counselors.

Section 504 of the Rehabilitation Act of 1973   Section 504 is part of a broad federal civil rights law regarding discrimination. According to Boyle and Weishaar (2001), Section 504 prohibits any public or private organization that receives federal funding "from discriminating against an *otherwise handicapped person* solely on the basis of a handicap" (p. 15; emphasis added). Additionally, Section 504 protects the rights of students with disabilities to a free and appropriate public education (FAPE; Thompson & Henderson, 2007). A student may be eligible for protection under Section 504 if he or she "(i) has a physical or mental impairment which substantially limits one or more such person's major life activities, (ii) has a record of such an impairment, or (iii) is regarded as having an impairment" (29 U.S.C § 706 [7] [6]). Typically, students are eligible for services under Section 504 if they have a medical condition (either permanent or temporary) such as diabetes, asthma, or confinement to a wheelchair; and/or are diagnosed with attention deficit hyperactivity disorder (ADHD), an alcohol or substance addiction, or behavior problems (Boyle & Weishaar, 2001).

T A B L E 9.1   Exceptional Education Terms, Acronyms, and Brief Definitions

Terms and Acronyms	Definitions
Accommodations	Deliberate procedures that support equal access to student instruction and assessment—designed to "level the playing field."
Adequate Yearly Progress (AYP)	An individual state's measure of yearly progress toward achieving statewide academic standards. "Adequate Yearly Progress" is the minimum level of improvement that states, school districts, and schools must achieve each year.
Americans with Disabilities Act of 1990 (ADA)	Civil rights legislation prohibiting discrimination against persons with disabilities in any setting.
Behavior Intervention Plan (BIP)	A plan designed to address student behavior problems, which may include positive behavior interventions and counseling services.
Child Study Team	A team of education professionals meeting and reviewing whether to evaluate a student for a potential disability.
Extended School Year Services (ESY)	Services provided to a student diagnosed with a disability beyond the normal school year, at no cost to the parents or caregivers.
Free Appropriate Public Education (FAPE)	Ensures that students diagnosed with a disability have an appropriate education that meets the student's unique educational needs at no expense to the parents or caregivers.
Functional Behavior Assessment (FBA)	A problem-solving process for addressing problematic student behavior.
Inclusion (Mainstreaming)	Students diagnosed with disabilities are fully integrated into the general population of students—conceptually related to least restrictive environment.
Independent Education Evaluation (IEE)	A parent's/caregiver's right to have their child re-evaluated for a disability by a professional outside the school system, which is paid for by the school.
Individual with Disabilities Education Improvement Act of 2004 (IDEIA)	Formerly known as the Education for All Handicap Children Act of 1975, Public Law 94–142. This law mandates that all students diagnosed with a disability receive free educational experiences designed to meet the particular needs of each student.

Individualized Education Program (IEP)	A written statement that is developed, reviewed, and revised as necessary, which describes the exceptional educational and related services specifically designed to meet the unique educational needs of a student with a disability.
Least Restrictive Environment (LRE)	A learning plan that recommends, to the maximum extent appropriate, that students diagnosed with disabilities are to be educated alongside students who are not disabled.
Language Learning Disability (LLD)	A disorder that may affect the comprehension and use of spoken or written language as well as nonverbal language, such as eye contact and tone of speech, in both adults and children.
Manifestation Determination	Prior to a student diagnosed with a disability being suspended from school for 10 days or more, the IEP team must meet to determine if the student's misbehavior was a function of his or her disability.
Office of Special Education Programs (OSEP)	An office of the U.S. Department of Education whose goal is to improve results for children with disabilities by providing leadership and financial support to assist states and local school districts.
Response to Intervention (RTI)	Response to Intervention is a process whereby Local Education Agencies (LEA; a public school, charter school, alternative school, etc.) delivering education to the student document a child's response to scientific, research-based intervention using a tiered approach. In contrast to the discrepancy criterion model, RTI provides early intervention for students experiencing difficulty learning. Read more: http://specialneedseducation.suite101.com/article.cfm/the_special_education_process#ixzz0TSkuldO4)
Specific Learning Disability (SLD or LD)	The official term used in federal legislation to refer to difficulty in certain areas of learning, rather than in all areas of learning. Synonymous with *learning disabilities*.
Section 504 of the Rehabilitation Act of 1973 (Section 504)	A civil rights act designed to protect the rights of individuals in places that receive federal funding, such as public schools.
Transition Services	Per IDEIA (2004), schools must provide services to students diagnosed with a disability to support their transition into the workforce, and specific provision must included in a student's IEPs if he or she is16 years old or older.
Triennial Reevaluation	Under IDEIA (2004), all students with an IEP must be reevaluated at least every three years to assess their placement and the appropriateness of services.

161

The Americans with Disabilities Act (ADA) of 1990.   ADA (1990) is a civil rights law that aligns with Section 504 in prohibiting discrimination against persons with disabilities. However, unlike Section 504, ADA is not limited to organizations receiving federal funding. More specifically, ADA prohibits discrimination of persons with disabilities in education, employment, public services, transportation, and telecommunications. It should be noted that both Section 504 and ADA afford the right to appropriate accommodation for persons with a disability, even if those persons do not qualify as eligible for exceptional education services (Cambron-McCabe, McCarthy, & Thomas, 2008).

Exceptional Education Legislation

The primary federal legislation regarding exceptional education for students with LDs is IDEIA (2004 [PL 108–146]). Initially passed as the Education of All Handicapped Children Act of 1975 (PL 94–142, 20 U.S.C. Section 1400 [d]), IDEIA addresses the historical practice of schools excluding and segregating students diagnosed with disabilities from their non-disabled peers (Turnbull, Stowe, & Huerta, 2007). Additionally, Turnbull and colleagues noted that the purpose of PL 94–142 was to assure the rights of all students diagnosed with a disability to a FAPE, to protect the rights of students diagnosed with a disability and their parents/caregivers to receive an appropriate education, to support state and local education systems in providing appropriate educational services to these students, and to hold state and local educational systems accountable for providing appropriate educational services to these students. PL 94–142 (1975) was amended by Congress in 1978 (Education Amendment of 1978 [PL 95–561]), 1983 (Education of the Handicapped Act Amendment of 1983 [PL 98–199]), 1986 (Handicapped Children's Protection Act [PL 98–372]), 1990 (Individuals with Disabilities Act [PL 101–476], 1997 (Individuals with Disabilities Act Education Amendment of 1997 [PL 105–17], and 2004 (IDEIA [PL 108–446]). Therefore, the primary exceptional education law for supporting students with LDs has evolved and has subsequently altered the role of professional school counselors in supporting students with disabilities and their families.

Unlike Section 504 and ADA (1990), IDEIA (2004) provided federal funding and requires states to guarantee a FAPE. FAPE is made available in the least restrictive environment (LRE) to students who necessitate exceptional education and related services as a result of a disability. According to IDEIA, students (ages 3 to 21) with an LD and who qualify for exceptional education services must be provided with individual educational services to support their development. Students qualify for IDEIA service if they are diagnosed with one of thirteen identified disabilities. Exceptional education services can significantly impact the academic performance of students with LDs. Table 9.2 presents the thirteen disability categories listed as handicapping conditions that may entitle a student to exceptional education services under IDEIA.

IDEIA (2004) also contains recent changes specific to students with LDs. These amendments include different ways to identify students with LDs, varying methods for providing early interventions, higher standards for hiring specialized

T A B L E 9.2   Thirteen Disability Conditions Listed under IDEIA (2004)

Disability Condition	Description
Autism	Developmental disability significantly affecting a student's verbal and nonverbal communication and social interactions, often evident by age three.
Deaf-blindness (DB)	Simultaneous hearing and visual impairments that cause significant communication and other developmental and education problems.
Deafness	A hearing impairment that is so significant that disables student's educational development and performance.
Emotional Disturbance (ED)	Student exhibits one or more of the following characteristics for a prolonged period, adversely affecting their educational performance: inability to learn that cannot be explained by intellectual, sensory, or health factors; inability to build and maintain satisfactory interpersonal relationships with peers and educators; inappropriate types of behavior or feelings under normal circumstances; a general, pervasive mood of unhappiness or depression; and a tendency to develop physical symptoms or fear in association with personal and school problems. The term does not apply to students who are socially maladjusted, unless it is determined that they are also emotionally disturbed.
Hearing Impairment (HI)	Impairment in a student's hearing, whether permanent or fluctuating, that adversely affects his or her educational performance.
Mental Retardation (MR)	The student scores at significantly sub-average levels of general intellectual functioning, existing concurrently with deficits in adaptive behavior.
Multiple Disabilities (MD)	Simultaneous impairments (i.e., mental retardation and blindness, mental retardation and orthopedic impairment, etc.), the combination of which causes significant educational needs that cannot be accommodated in an exceptional educational program designed to address only one of the disabilities.
Orthopedic Impairment (OI)	A significant orthopedic impairment, such as nonambulatory cerebral palsy, that adversely affects a student's educational performance.

(Continued)

T A B L E 9.2   Thirteen Disability Conditions Listed under IDEIA (2004) (Continued)

Disability Condition	Description
Other Health Impairment (OHI)	The student has limited strength, vitality, or alertness, including a heightened alertness to environmental stimuli which results in limited alertness with respect to the educational environment. OHI can be the result of chronic or acute health problems and adversely affects his or her educational performance.
Specific Learning Disability (LD)	A disorder in one or more of the psychological processes involved in using language or understanding, spoken or written, that may manifest in an imperfect ability to listen, think, speak, read, write, spell, or do mathematic calculations.
Speech or Language Impairment (SI)	Communication disorder such as stuttering, impaired articulation, a language impairment, or a voice impairment that adversely affects a student's educational performance.
Traumatic Brain Injury (TBI)	Acquired injury to the brain caused by an external physical force, resulting in total or partial functional disability or psychosocial impairment, or both, which adversely affects a student's educational performance.
Visual Impairment including Blindness (VI)	Impairment in vision that, even with correction, adversely affects a student's educational performance.

NOTE: Adapted from the National Dissemination Center for Children with Disabilities. (2009, April). *Categories of disabilities under IDEA*. Washington, DC: Author.

teachers working with this exceptionality, more flexible discipline policies, and specific consequences for students based on individual school decisions (CEC, 2007b). IDEIA also provides for specific changes to IEPs, allowing for more specific and accountable goals and objectives that reflect the individual student with an LD and facilitate progress. Success for the student with a learning disability requires a focus on individual achievement, progress, and learning (Cortiella, 2006).

Diagnosing a Learning Disability under IDEIA (2004)

IDEIA (2004, n.p.; see summary in Kavale et al., 2009) stated that an LD is "A disorder in one or more of the basic psychological processes involved in understanding or in using language, spoken or written, which disorder may manifest itself in the imperfect ability to listen, speak, read, write, spell, or do mathematics calculations" (p. 40). Students with LDs must have at least average cognitive or intellectual potential as measured by a standard intelligence test (e.g., Wechsler Intelligence Scale for Children—4th ed. [Wechsler, 2001]), yet their achievement in one or more academic areas must be significantly below their measured ability.

Typically, there appears to be an inconsistency between the student's potential (aptitude/ability) and his or her actual achievement. According to the National Center for Learning Disabilities (NCLD, 2001), "LD is not a single disorder. It is a term that refers to a group of disorders" (p. 1). Table 9.3 presents the different disabilities within the category of LDs.

Students with LDs require tailored support services. According to LDA (2004c), each person with an LD is unique and experiences different degrees of challenges. However, NICHCY (2004) suggested that a common characteristic among students with LDs is uneven areas of ability. For example, a student with dyscalculia (problems with arithmetic and math concepts) may be very able in the domains of reading, writing, and spelling. Assouline, Nicpon, and Huber (2006) noted that students with LDs might also be classified as dual exceptionality, being identified as gifted/talented in one or more areas while also possessing an LD in another area. It is essential to remember that each student with an LD has varying abilities and needs.

Recall that the definition of an LD does not include processing problems primarily caused by visual, hearing, or motor disabilities. However, students with exceptional education diagnoses of Visual Impaired, Hearing Impaired, and Physically Impaired may also have learning disorders (Horowitz, 2005). Additionally, LDA (2004c) suggested that an LD "cannot be cured or fixed; it is a lifelong challenge" (p. 1). Readers may wish to refer to Ahearn (2009) for an overview of the changes in state eligibility requirements for diagnoses of specific learning disabilities.

Response to Intervention (RTI) in Diagnosing Learning Disabilities   In the IDEIA (2004) there are new perspectives for exploring the different ways of identifying an LD (CEC, 2007b; Kavale et al. 2009). More specifically, IDEIA offers additional means for diagnosing students with learning differences that

T A B L E 9.3   Disabilities and Disorders within Specific Learning Disabilities

Technical Name	Common Name	Descriptors
Dyslexia	Learning disabilities in reading	Difficulties with processing language, reading, writing, and spelling
Dyscalculia	Learning disabilities in mathematics	Difficulties with mathematics skills and computation
Dysgraphia	Learning disabilities in writing	Difficulties with handwriting, spelling, and composition
Dyspraxia	Disorder in the areas of fine motor skill development	Difficulties with coordination and manual dexterity
Information Processing Disorder—Central Auditory Processing Disorder	Disorder in interpreting auditory information	Difficulties with language development and reading
Information Processing Disorder—Visual Processing Disorder	Disorder in interpreting visual information	Difficulties with reading, writing, and mathematics
Information Processing Disorder—Attention Deficit Hyperactivity Disorder (ADHD)	Disorder in concentration and focus	Difficulties with impulsivity, distractibility, and hyperactivity

NOTE: Adapted from the National Center for Learning Disabilities (NCLD), www.ncld.org.

move away from the traditional requirement of a significant intelligence-achievement discrepancy. The RTI is an approach to help determine eligibility based on student responses to research-based interventions (Gresham, 2009). The NCLD (2006) defined RTI as "a comprehensive, multi-step process that closely monitors how the student is responding to different types of services and instruction" (p. 12). Typically, RTI employs a three-tier approach; however, some school districts may utilize a four-tier model where exceptional education referral begins at the final tier (Trolley, Haas, & Patti, 2009).

RTI utilizes district-approved strategies not otherwise used in the classroom. Some of these could be specialized reading programs, pull-out math groups, or one-on-one reading comprehension assistance. Although RTI may allow each state to develop their own criteria for what qualifies students for eligibility for the diagnosis of a LD (Zirkel & Krohn, 2008), it cannot be used as the sole approach when determining which students are eligible for an LD diagnosis and other special education services (Gresham, 2009). There are still many questions about the efficiency and effectiveness of using the RTI criteria model (Kavale & Spaulding, 2008), and there is limited evidence of RTI models that include the services of a school counselor. Regardless, RTI is currently being implemented

TABLE 9.4   The Three-Tier Approach of RTI as Relates to Professional School Counseling Services

Tier	Tier Name	Description	School Counseling Services
1	Screening and Group Intervention	Involves all students via traditional educational services, where some students are identified as "at-risk" and may require supplemental services.	Coordination and facilitation of a comprehensive developmental school counseling program for all students.
2	Targeted Interventions	Typically involves about 20% of those students who require more intense interventions in order to make adequate progress.	More focused school counseling services such as tailored group and individual counseling, and consultation.
3	Intensive, Systemic Interventions and Comprehensive Evaluation	Typically involves 1% to 5% of students who require individualized and intensive interventions in order to address skills deficits. Students who are not responsive to these interventions are eligible for services under IDEIA (2004).	Focused school counseling services such as consistent and individualized counseling and consultation services. Often, students at this tier are receiving multiple school counseling intervention strategies.

NOTE: Adapted from the National Center for Learning Disabilities (NCLD), www.ncld.org.

as a part of IDEIA (CEC, 2007b). The American School Counselor Association (ASCA; 2008) advocated that professional school counselors work to "identify struggling students and collaborate with other educators to provide appropriate interventions through the RTI process" (p. 2). For elaboration of the RTI three-tier approach and school counseling service delivery, see Table 9.4.

RECOMMENDATIONS FOR SCHOOL COUNSELING PRACTICE

Research supports the belief that students with LDs are at risk for adverse academic, social-emotional, and vocational consequences (e.g., Kaffenberger & Seligman, 2007; Kemp, Segal, & Cutter, 2009; Shechtman & Katz, 2007). This section reviews the behavioral cues of students with LDs that may be observed by educators and school counselors.

General Intervention Strategies

ASCA (2005) advocated that professional school counselors work to support the academic, vocational, and personal/social development of all their students.

Moreover, ASCA (2004) stated that school counselors should advocate for students with LDs and provide comprehensive school counseling services including providing group and individual counseling, assisting with designing and implementing accommodation plans and modifications, advocating for students and families, providing collaboration as part of the comprehensive school program, assisting in middle-to-high-school transition planning, working on a multidisciplinary team that identifies students who may need assessments to determine special needs, and serving as consultants for parents and caregivers, teachers, and administrators. However, the ASCA (2004) also noted that "it is inappropriate for the professional school counselor to serve in supervisory or administrative roles" (p. 1) regarding IEPs and 504 plans. Volker and Ray (2006) suggested however that school counselors work from a systemic perspective when assisting students with special needs and their families.

Systemic Collaborative Consultants   In supporting students with LDs, professional school counselors must serve as systemic, collaborative consultants with all stakeholders (Volker & Ray, 2006). According to Myers (2005), school counselors need to collaborate with professionals both inside (e.g., teachers, administration, school psychologists, behavioral specialists, and school social workers) and outside of schools (families, physicians, and mental health professionals) to gain fresh perspectives. Collaborative consultation can assist counselors in providing effective services to students with LDs and their families. See Table 9.5 for additional resources.

First, as a collaborative consultant, professional school counselors need to serve as educators in their work with students, parents and caregivers, and school administrators and staff (Allen, 2001). Counselors need to educate students on what it means to be a person with an LD and assist them in developing methods to talk with others about their disability. Additionally, parents and caregivers must be educated on how to speak with their student about his or her LD, and

T A B L E 9.5   Additional Web Resources

American School Counselor Association (ASCA)	www.schoolcounselor.org
Council for Exceptional Children (CEC)	www.cec.sped.org
Family Center for Technology and Disabilities	www.fctd.info
Family Resource Center on Disabilities	www.frcd.org
International Dyslexia Association	www.interdys.org
LDOnline (Web site on learning disabilities)	www.ldonline.org
Learning Disabilities Association of America (LDA)	www.ldaamerica.org
National Center for Learning Disabilities (NCLD)	www.ld.org
National Center for Special Education Personnel and Related Service Providers	www.personnelcenter.org
National Information Center for Children and Youth with Disabilities	www.nichcy.org

counselors should direct them to available resources in the community that may serve as support systems (Bergin & Bergin, 2001). Within a comprehensive school counseling program (ASCA, 2005), education may also include conducting parenting seminars on practical strategies for supporting students with LDs. Additionally, school counselors should provide teachers with resources for supporting both their teaching and students' social skills development (see Ruegg [2006] for social skills strategies counselors can train classroom teachers in to support students with LDs). Finally, counselors must educate other educators about their views and beliefs about students with LDs in their classrooms—modeling to other educators that *all* students are worthy of an educator's individualized attention (Lambie, 2004).

School counselors are often asked to serve as collaborative consultants when planning modifications and goals for students with LDs (IEPs). Kampwirth (2006) suggested some consultative strategies for counselors in promoting a positive IEP implementation. These collaborative, consultative services include modifying the curriculum to adapt to a student's learning style, utilizing cooperative groups and peer involvement, communicating concerns and progress with the student's parents and caregivers, and encouraging specific activities to get parents and caregivers involved in their student's learning experience. Additionally, Milsom and Harley (2005) noted that school counselors should serve as consultants when supporting students with LDs transition in to the workforce or post-secondary education or training. Further, Milson and Harley advocated that counselors provide resources to parents and caregivers to help them support their student's success; such resources may focus on the student's time management, organization, and study and note-taking skills (for elaboration of these recommendations, please consult Milsom & Harley).

Another collaborative, consultative strategy counselors may employ in supporting students with LDs is bibliotherapy (Jack & Ronan, 2008). Bibliotherapy is suggested as a collaborative, consultative approach (rather than individual counseling) for two primary reasons: the most influential contributor to student's academic achievement is family engagement in a student's educational experience (Davis & Lambie, 2005), and students with LDs may have difficulty reading; therefore, counselors should involve parents and caregivers in the bibliotherapy process with their student. Sridhar and Vaughn (2000) concluded that bibliotherapy increases self-esteem and reading comprehension in students with LDs. In addition, bibliotherapy was found to be effective in improving students' attitudes, self-understanding, and confidence. Further, Forgan (2000) found that bibliotherapy was an effective tool in teaching students new problem solving strategies. Research also shows that bibliotherapy can be an effective strategy for supporting students with learning differences, as long as the reading material is appropriate to the student's level of comprehension and vocabulary (Bergin & Bergin, 2001).

Counselors should also serve as collaborative consultants in their delivery of classroom guidance curriculum. Horowitz (2007) underscored the importance of social-emotional skills development for students with LDs, and the need for educators to foster the development of these skills in these young people. For example, Horowitz suggested that educators identify and acknowledge students' competencies and personal resources while recognizing opportunities to reinforce these strengths and identify "teachable moments" (Johns, Crowley, & Guetzloe, 2005, p. 4). Additionally, professional school counselors may also facilitate social skills training experiences by providing collaborative groups. To review the role of professional school counselors in training teachers to teach social skills, please consult Johns et al.

Counseling Services

Research supports that students with LDs need additional social-emotional support, which may come in the form of counseling service facilitated by school counselors. As noted in IDEIA (2004), "related services" includes counseling services for students with learning disabilities. According to Cambron-McCabe and colleagues (2008), counseling services should be included in a student's IEP when he or she requires such services to support the learning process, and the services are provided by a qualified helping professional (professional school counselor). Consequently, counselors should provide counseling, both individual and group, along with the collaborative consultation services reviewed above, to students with LDs.

The professional school counselor should also be doing some individual counseling with students with special needs. Traditionally, students with LDs receive behavioral modifications, academic skills development interventions, and other forms of educational remediation per their IEP; however, "their emotional difficulties have been largely ignored" (Shechtman & Pastor, 2005, p. 322). Limited research has been published on the outcomes of counseling interventions with this student-client population (Pattison, 2005). Recent research has emerged which offers promise for school counselors working with students with LDs.

Students with LDs can experience significant problems in their interpersonal relationships. Research supports that students with LDs have a lower quality of friendships, lack trust in self or in others, and often score high on levels of loneliness and peer rejection (Al-Yagon, 2007). Shechtman and Katz (2007) noted that students with LDs have lower security attachments than their non-disabled peers, negatively contributing to the student's already-impaired ability to establish functional interpersonal relationships (friendships). Shechtman and Pastor (2005) stated that anxious and lonely students "need to reexperience positive interpersonal relationships" (p. 323), and the success of the counselor-student alliance has been found to be the strongest predictor of positive counseling outcomes (Shechtman & Katz). Further, when comparing the outcomes of cognitive-behavioral and humanistic counseling groups with children with LDs, Shechtman and Pastor found that the humanistic approach was more effective. Therefore, based on the research and these students' needs, a humanistic counseling approach is suggested to support students with LDs.

A humanistic counseling approach (Rogers, 1995) advocates that a counselor should empathize with his or her students' experiences of their world while providing a safe environment that supports the students' intrinsic abilities to grow and develop. This therapeutic relationship experience will contribute to the student's ability to more effectively cope with the problems they are currently facing as well as future challenges. Humanistic counselors are congruent and genuine, and express unconditional positive regard and empathy to their students. Miller, Taylor and West (1980) found that empathy had the strongest effect on clients' positive behavioral changes, where the counselor expresses unconditional positive regard and relatedness. Within a humanistic counseling approach, the counselor focuses on process (the development of a safe, trusting therapeutic relationship) rather than content (problem-solving). As Schechtman and Katz (2007) noted, before a person can have functional interpersonal relationships, he or she must develop trust in himself or herself and others. The development of a humanistic counseling relationship can promote this trust.

A review of all the theoretical tenets and therapeutic strategies of a humanistic counseling approach to support students with LDs is beyond the scope of this chapter. However, it is recommended that readers consult Williams and Lair (1991) and Rogers (1995) for elaboration. Additionally, to review counseling approaches grounded in humanistic theory, readers may wish to consult Smith (2005), a solution-focused brief counseling approach for supporting students with LDs, and Lambie and Milsom (in press), a narrative counseling approach for supporting students diagnosed with LDs.

Group Counseling   Group counseling is an effective intervention strategy for supporting students with LDs (Packman & Bratton, 2003; Shechtman & Pastor, 2005) and a primary service of the ASCA (2005) *National Model*©. Milsom (2006) suggested that school counselors provide counseling groups that promote cooperative behaviors as well as strengthen tolerance and respect for differences. Packman and Bratton found school-based group play therapy interventions grounded in humanistic principles to be effective in decreasing students with LDs problematic behavior. Additionally, Shechtman and Pastor found group counseling based on humanistic tenets to be effective in improving the academic achievement of students with LDs (even more effective than a cognitive-behavioral group). Therefore, group counseling strategies based on humanistic principles are suggested for professional school counselors working with students with LDs.

Group counseling strategies for students with LDs should be developmentally appropriate and match the group participants' needs. Bergin and Bergin (2001) suggested that school counselors facilitating counseling groups for students with LDs use both concrete and visual strategies. For example, the counselor may model appropriate behavior and have the group participants role-play the desired behaviors and communication. Additionally, counselors may use other concrete and tangible counseling activities with students with LDs, such as drawing, flow charts, dry erase boards, feeling charts, and games (e.g., *Ungame Teen Card Game*). Counseling groups for school-age students need to be engaging, small (three to eight participants), action-orientated, and personally relevant to each of the students. Packman and Bratton (2003) and McEachern (2004) recommended play, art, music, and expressive art therapeutic counseling strategies for school counselors working with students with LDs. School counseling groups for students with LDs may include social skills groups, friendship groups, stress management groups, self-esteem groups, anger management groups, and academic success and achievement groups. It is recommended that interested readers consult Greenberg (2003) and Brigman and Earley (2008) for specific school-based group counseling activities.

SUMMARY

All students should receive comprehensive school counseling services (ASCA, 2005); however, some student subpopulations that have been identified as at high risk for negative academic, social-emotional, and vocational success and who have been historically marginalized and discriminated against (students with LDs), require additional school-based counseling services. This chapter offered professional school counselors an introduction to the educational and civil rights statutes relating to persons with disabilities, reviewed common challenges that students with LDs struggle with, and presented school-based intervention approaches that have been found effective in supporting these students. However, as also noted, all students with learning disabilities are unique and experience different struggles, necessitating intervention strategies tailored to each student's individual needs.

Professional school counselors are educational specialists with unique graduate-level preparation, who are trained as advocates and agents for systemic change to support all students' achievements and success (ASCA, 2005). They are especially concerned with those students whose voice has been marginalized and kept silent. As systemic, collaborative consultants and humanistic counselors, the professional school counselor is well positioned to support the holistic needs of students with LDs. However, the legal statutes and the research relating to students with LDs continues to evolve; therefore, it is recommended that readers regularly consult with the Council for Exceptional Children (www.cec.sped. org/), the Learning Disabilities Association of America (www.ldaamerica.org), and the National Center for Learning Disabilities (www.ld.org) to update their knowledgebase and ability to ethically and effectively serve these students.

REFERENCES

Ahearn, E. M. (2009). State eligibility requirements for specific learning disabilities. *Communication Disorders Quarterly, 30*, 120–128.

Allen, J. (2001). Counseling the special needs student. In D. S. Sandhu (Ed.). *Elementary school counseling in the new millennium* (pp. 173–181). Alexandria, VA: American Counseling Association.

Al-Yagon, M. (2007). Socioemotional and behavioral adjustment among school-aged children with learning disabilities: The moderating role of material personal resources. *Journal of Special Education, 40*, 205–217.

American School Counselor Association. (2008). *Position statement: The professional school counselor and response to intervention.* Retrieved June 9, 2009, from http://asca2. timberlakepublishing.com//files/PS_Intervention.pdf

American School Counselor Association. (2005). *The ASCA national model: A framework for school counseling programs* (2nd ed.). Alexandria, VA: Author.

American School Counselor Association. (2004). *Position statement: Special-needs students: The professional school counselor and students with special needs.* Retrieved June 8, 2009, from http://asca2.timberlakepublishing.com//files/Special%20Needs.pdf

Americans with Disabilities Act of 1990 (PL 101–336), 42 U.S.C.Secs. 12101 *et seq.*

Assouline, S. G., Nicpon, M. F., & Huber, D. H. (2006). The impact of vulnerabilities and strengths on the academic experiences of twice-exceptional students: A message to school counselors. *Professional School Counseling, 10,* 14–24.

Bergin, J., & Bergin, J. (2001). Counseling children with learning disabilities. In D. S. Sandhu (Ed.), *Elementary school counseling in the new millennium* (pp. 183–191). Alexandria, VA: American Counseling Association.

Boyle, J. R., & Weishaar, M. (2001). *Special education law with cases.* Needham Heights, MA: Allyn & Bacon.

Brigman, G., & Earley, B. (2008). *Group counseling for school counselors: A practical guide* (3rd ed.). Portland, ME: Walch Publishing.

Cambron-McCabe, N. H., Thomas, S. B., & McCarthy, M. M. (2008). *Public school law: Teachers' and students' rights* (6th ed.). Boston, MA: Allyn & Bacon.

Cortiella, C. (2006). *NCLB and IDEA: What parents of students with disabilities need to know and do.* Minneapolis, MN: University of Minnesota, National Center on Educational Outcomes.

Council for Exceptional Children. (2007a). *Learning disabilities.* Retrieved June 8, 2009, from http://www.cec.sped.org/AM/Template.cfm?Section=Learning_Disabilities& Template=/TaggedPage/TaggedPageDisplay.cfm&TPLID=37&ContentID=5629

Council for Exceptional Children. (2007b). *A primer on the IDEA 2004 regulations.* Retrieved June 8, 2009, from http://www.cec.sped.org/AM/Template.cfm? Section=Home&TEMPLATE=/CM/ContentDisplay.cfm&CONTENTID=7839

Davis, K. M., & Lambie, G. W. (2005). Family engagement: A collaborative, systemic approach for middle school counselors. *Professional School Counseling, 9,* 144–151.

Education for All Handicapped Children Act of 1975 (PL 94–142), 20 U.S.C. 1400 *et seq.*

Forgan, J. W. (2002). Using bibliotherapy to teach problem solving. *Intervention in School and Clinic, 38*(2), 75–89.

Goldstein, S., & Schwebach, A. (2009). Neurological basis of learning disabilities. In C. R. Reynolds, & E. Fletcher-Janzen (Eds.), *Handbook of clinical child neuropsychology* (pp. 187–202). New York: Springer.

Greenberg, K. R. (2003). *Group counseling in K–12 schools: A handbook for school counselors.* Boston, MA: Pearson Education.

Gresham, F. M. (2009). Using response to intervention for identification of specific learning disabilities. In A. Akin-Little, S. G. Little, M. A. Bray, T. J. Kehle (Eds.), *Behavioral interventions in schools: Evidence-based positive strategies* (pp. 205–220). Washington, DC: American Psychological Association.

Heinrichs, R. R. (2003). A whole-schoolapproach to bullying: Special considerations for children with exceptionalities. *Intervention in School and Clinic, 38,* 195–204.

Horowitz, S. H. (2005). Learning disabilities: What they are, and what they are not. *Children's Voices, 14*(6). Retrieved June 8, 2009, from http://www.cwla.org/voice/ 0512voice.htm

Horowitz, S. H. (2007). *How does it feel? The social/emotional side of LD*. Retrieved June 8, 2009, from http://www.ncld.org/idex2.php?option=com_content&task=view&id=1340&pop=1&page=0

Individuals with Disabilities Education Improvement Act of 2004 (P.L.108–446), 20 U.S.C. 1400 *et seq.*

Jack, S. J., & Ronan, K. R. (2008). Bibliotherapy: Practice and research. *School Psychology International, 29*, 161–182.

Johns, B. H., Crowley, E. P., & Guetzloe, E. (2005). The central role of teaching social skills. *Focus on Exceptional Children, 37*, 1–8.

Kaffenberger, C., & Seligman, L. (2007). Helping students with mental and emotional disorders. In B.T. Erford (Ed.), *Transforming the school counseling profession* (2nd ed., pp. 351–383). Upper Saddle River, NJ: Merrill Prentice Hall.

Kampwirth, T. J. (2006). *Collaborative consultation in the schools: Effective practices for students with learning and behavior problems* (3rd ed.). Upper Saddle River, NJ: Pearson Prentice Hall.

Kavale, K. A., & Spaulding, L. S. (2008). Is Response to Intervention good policy for specific learning disability? *Learning Disabilities Research & Practice, 23*, 169–179.

Kavale, K. A., Spaulding, L. S., & Beam, A. P. (2009). A time to define: Making the specific learning disability definition prescribe *specific* learning disability. *Learning Disability Quarterly, 32*, 39–48.

Kemp, J., Segal, J., & Cutter, D. (2007). *Learning disabilities in children: Learning disability symptoms, types, and testing*. Retrieved June 8, 2009, from http://www.helpguide.org/mental/learning_disabilities.htm

Kortering, L. J., & Christenson, S. (2009). Engaging students in school and learning: The real deal for school completion. *Exceptionality, 17*, 5–15.

Lambie, G. W. (2004). Motivational enhancement therapy: A tool for professional school counselors working with adolescents. *Professional School Counseling, 7*, 268–276.

Lambie, G. W., & Williamson, L. L. (2004). The challenge to change from guidance counseling to professional school counseling: A historical proposition. *Professional School Counseling, 8*, 124–131.

Lambie, G. W., & Milsom, A. (in press). A narrative approach to supporting students diagnosed with learning disabilities. *Journal of Counseling & Development.*

Learning Disabilities Association of America. (2004a). *Types of learning disabilities*. Retrieved June 8, 2009, from http://www.ldaamerica.org/aboutld/parents/ld_basics/types.asp

Learning Disabilities Association of America. (2004b). For teachers. Retrieved June 8, 2009, from http://www.ldaamerica.org/aboutld/teachers/index.asp

Learning Disabilities Association of America. (2004c). *Learning disabilities: Signs, symptoms and strategies*. Retrieved June 8, 2009, from http://www.ldaamerica.org/aboutld/teachers/understanding/print_ld.asp

McEachern, A. G. (2004). Students with learning disabilities: Counseling issues and strategies. In B. T. Erford (Ed.), *Professional school counseling: A handbook.* (pp. 591–600). Austin, TX: ProEd.

Medina, C., & Luna, G. (2004). Learning at the margins. *Rural Special Education Quarterly, 23*(4), 10–16.

Meltzer, L., Katzie-Cohen, T. Miller, L., & Roditi, B. (2001). The impact of effort and strategy used on academic performance: Student and teacher perceptions. *Learning Disabilities Quarterly, 34,* 85–99.

Miller, W., Taylor, C., & West, J. (1980). Focused versus broad spectrum behavior therapy for problem drinkers. *Journal of Consulting and Clinical Psychology, 48,* 590–601.

Milsom, A., & Hartley, M. T. (2005). Assisting students with learning disabilities transitioning to college: What school counselors should know? *Professional School Counseling, 8,* 436–441.

Myers, H. N. (2005). How elementary school counselors can meet the needs for students with disabilities. *Professional School Counseling, 8,* 442–450.

National Center for Learning Disabilities. (2006, April). *IDEA parent guide: A comprehensive guide to your rights and responsibilities under the Individual with Disabilities Education Act (IDEA 2004).* New York: Author. Retrieved June 8, 2009, from http://www.eric.ed.gov/ERICDocs/data/ericdocs2sql/content_ storage_01/0000019b/80/28/05/9a.pdf

National Center for Learning Disabilities. (2001). *LD at a glance.* New York: Author.

National Dissemination Center for Children with Disabilities. (2009, April). *Categories of disabilities under IDEA.* Washington, DC: Author.

National Dissemination Center for Children with Disabilities. (2004, January). *Learning disabilities: Disabilities fact sheet—No. 7.* Washington, DC: Author.

National Information Center for Children and Youth with Disabilities. (2004, February). *Briefing paper: Reading and learning disabilities* (4th ed.) Washington, DC: Author.

National Research Center on Learning Disabilities. (2007). *And Miles to Go…: State SLD requirements and authoritative recommendations.* Retrieved June 7, 2009, from http://www.nrcld.org/about/research/states/section7.html

Packman, J. & Bratton, S. C. (2003). A school-based group play/activity therapy intervention with learning disabled preadolescents exhibiting behavior problems. *International Journal of Play Therapy, 12*(2), 7–29.

Pattison, S. (2005). Making a difference for young people with learning disabilities: A model for inclusive counseling practice. *Counseling and Psychotherapy Research, 5,* 120–130.

Putnam, M. L. (2007). Crisis intervention with adolescents with learning disabilities. In J. Carlson & J. Lewis (Eds.), *Counseling the adolescent: Individual, family, school interventions* (5th ed., pp. 61–104). Denver, CO: Love Publishing.

Rock, E., & Leff, E. H. (2007). The professional school counselor and students with disabilities. In B. T. Erford (Ed.), *Transforming the school counseling profession* (2nd ed., pp. 318–250). Upper Saddle River, NJ: Merrill Prentice Hall.

Rodis, P. (2001). Forging identities, tackling problems, and arguing with culture: Psychotherapy with persons who have learning disabilities. In P. Rodis, A. Garrod, & M. L. Boscardin (Eds.), *Learning disabilities & life stories* (pp. 205–230). Boston: Allyn & Bacon.

Rogers, C. R. (1995). *A way of being.* New York: Houghton Mifflin Company.

Romano, D. M. (2006). *The impact of preparation, field experience and personal awareness on counselors' attitudes toward providing services to Section 504 students with learning disabilities.* Unpublished University of New Orleans dissertation.

Retrieved June 7, 2009, from http://proquest.umi.com/pqdlink?Ver=1&Exp=06-07-2014&FMT=7&DID=1192188001&RQT=309&attempt=1&cfc=1

Ruegg, E. (2006). Social skills in children with learning disabilities: Using psychotherapy in the classroom. *Annuals of the American Psychotherapy Association, 9*(3), 14–21.

Schmidt, J. J. (2008). *Counseling in schools: Comprehensive programs of responsive services for all students* (5th ed.). Boston: Pearson Education.

Section 504 of the Rehabilitation Act of 1973 (PL 93–651), 29 U.S.C. 794, Sec. 504, 34 C.F.R. 104–104.61.

Shechtman, Z., & Katz, E. (2007). Therapeutic bonding in group as an explanatory variable of progress in the social competence of students with learning disabilities. *Group dynamics: Theory, research, and practice, 11,* 117–128.

Shechtman, Z., & Pastor, R. (2005). Cognitive-behavioral and humanistic group treatment for children with learning disabilities: A comparison of outcome and process. *Journal of Counseling Psychology, 52,* 322–336.

Smith, I. C. (2005). Solution-focused brief therapy with people with learning disabilities: A case study. *British Journal of Learning Disabilities, 33,* 102–105.

Sridhar, D., & Vaughn, S. (2000). Bibliotherapy for all. *Teaching Exceptional Children, 33*(2), 74–84.

Steedly, K. M., Schwartz, A., Levin, M., & Luke, S. D. (2008). *Social skills and academic achievement.* Evidence of Education 3(2), Retrieved June 9, 2009, from http://www.nichcy.org/InformationResources/Documents/NICHCY%20PUBS/NICHCY_EE_Social_skills.pdf

Thompson, C. L., & Henderson, D. A. (2007). *Counseling children.* Belmont, CA: Thomas Brooks/Cole.

Trolley, B. C., Haas, H. S., & Patti, D. C. (2009). *The school counselor's guide to special education.* Thousand Oaks, CA: Corwin Press.

US Department of Education, Office of Special Education and Rehabilitation Services, Office of Special Education Programs. (2006). *Twenty-sixth annual (2004) report to congress on the implementation of the Individuals with Disabilities Education Act (Vol. 2).* Washington, DC: Author.

Valente, W. D., & Valente, C. M. (2001). *Law in the Schools* (5th ed.). Upper Saddle River, NJ: Prentice Hall

Vernon, A. (2009). *Counseling children & adolescents* (4th ed.). Denver, CO: Love Publishing.

Volker, T., & Ray, K. E. (2006). Counseling exceptional individuals and their families: A systems perspective. *Professional School Counseling, 10,* 58–65.

Wechsler, D. (2001). *Wechsler Intelligence Scale for Children* (4th ed.). San Antonio, TX: Psychological Corporation.

Willliams, W. C., & Lair, G. S. (1991). Using a person-centered approach with children who have a disability. *Elementary School Guidance & Counseling, 25,* 194–204.

Witherell, C. S., & Rodis, P. (2001). "Shimmers of delight and intellect:" Building learning communities of promise and possibility. In P. Rodis, A. Garrod, & M. L. Boscardin (Eds.), *Learning disabilities & life stories* (pp. 165–176). Boston: Allyn & Bacon.

Zirkel, P. A., & Krohn, N. (2008). RTI after IDEA. *Teaching Exceptional Children, 40,* 71–73.

Short Biographies of Contributors

CHAPTER 1: ATTENTION DEFICIT HYPERACTIVITY DISORDER

Dr. Linda Webb is an assistant professor in the Department of Counselor Education at Florida Atlantic University. She has been a kindergarten and second grade teacher, and has worked with students as a school counselor at the elementary and high school levels. As part of her research interests, Dr. Webb has been involved in the co-development of and research evaluating the effectiveness of the Student Success Skills (SSS) program aimed at helping students improve learning, social, and self-management skills associated with school success. She also provides training to school counselors across the country in SSS implementation and program evaluation. Dr. Webb's interest in program development aimed at helping students improve school performance extends to a school counselor intervention program targeting students with ADHD.

CHAPTER 2: EXTERNALIZING BEHAVIOR DISORDERS: SUPPORTING STUDENTS WITH AGGRESSION AND VIOLENT TENDENCIES

Dr. Kerry Bernes is an associate professor of Educational and Counselling Psychology at the University of Lethbridge in Lethbridge, Alberta, Canada. He is also a Registered Psychologist in Alberta and board certified in Clinical Psychology by the American Board of Professional Psychology. Dr. Bernes also spent eight years on the Calgary Board of Education.

Ms. Jennifer Bernes is a registered psychologist working in private practice in Lethbridge, Alberta, Canada. She has worked extensively in assessing and treating violent youth in a Secure Treatment facility in Canada.

CHAPTER 3: INTERNALIZING BEHAVIOR DISORDERS: SUPPORTING STUDENTS WITH DEPRESSION, ANXIETY, AND SELF-INJURIOUS BEHAVIOR

Christopher A. Sink, Ph.D., NCC, LMHC, professor of Counselor Education at Seattle Pacific University (15+ years), has been actively involved with the school counseling profession for nearly 30 years. Prior to serving as a counselor educator, he worked as a secondary and post-secondary school counselor. He has published extensively in the areas of school counseling, promoting comprehensive school counseling, achievement, and spirituality. He has served as editor of the journals *Professional School Counsel* (ASCA) and *Counseling and Values* (ACA).

CHAPTER 4: EATING DISORDERS, OBESITY, AND BODY IMAGE CONCERNS: PREVENTION AND INTERVENTION

Angela D. Bardick, B.F.A., B.Ed., M.Ed., is a registered psychologist in Alberta, Canada who specializes in the prevention and treatment of eating disorders, obesity, and body image concerns. Prior to becoming a psychologist, she worked for five years as an elementary school teacher.

Shelly Russell–Mayhew, Ph.D., is an assistant professor of applied psychology in the Faculty of Education, University of Calgary, Alberta, Canada. Her research interests include the prevention of weight-related issues such as eating disorders, obesity, and body image issues, and the development and evaluation of school-based resources such as school-based mental health, comprehensive school health programming, and inter-professional practice.

Kerry Bernes, Ph.D., is an associate professor of Educational and Counselling Psychology at the University of Lethbridge in Lethbridge, Alberta, Canada. He is also a Registered Psychologist in Alberta and he is board certified in Clinical Psychology by the American Board of Professional Psychology. Dr. Bernes also spent 8 years on the Calgary Board of Education.

Ms. Jennifer Bernes is a registered psychologist working in private practice in Lethbridge, Alberta, Canada. She has worked extensively in assessing and treating violent youth in a Secure Treatment facility in Canada.

CHAPTER 5: SUBSTANCE ABUSE: IMPLICATIONS FOR SCHOOL COUNSELING PRACTICE

Glenn W. Lambie, Ph.D., LPC, NCC, NCSC, CCMHC, is an associate professor and school counseling coordinator in the Counselor Education Program at the University of Central Florida. He earned his Master's degree in Counselor Education from Virginia Commonwealth University, an advanced certificate in Professional Counseling from the Medical College of Virginia/ VCU, and a doctoral degree in Counselor Education from The College of William & Mary. Dr. Lambie has worked in the counseling profession for 15 years as a counselor educator, professional school counselor, and family and individual therapist. He has published significantly in the areas of professional school counseling, counselor development and supervision, and counseling children and adolescent "at-risk" populations. Dr. Lambie has served on the ASCA Ethics Committee and on the editorial boards of *Professional School Counseling* (ASCA) and the *Journal of Counseling and Development* (ACA).

CHAPTER 6: SEXUAL ISSUES

Carolyn Stone, Ed.D., is a professor of Counselor Education at the University of North Florida, where she teaches and conducts research on the use of data and legal and ethical issues for student service personnel. Prior to becoming a counselor educator, Stone spent 22 years with the Duval County Public School District in Jacksonville, Florida as a school counselor and Supervisor of Guidance over 225 counselors. Stone was the American School Counselor Association's (ASCA) President in 2006 and is in her seventh year on ASCA's Ethics Committee. Stone is a past President of the Florida Counseling Association and the Florida Association of Counselor Educators and Supervisors. Stone is a sought-after presenter and has delivered over 400 keynote speeches and workshops in 48 states and 14 countries.

CHAPTER 7: STUDENTS WITH SEVERE ACTING-OUT BEHAVIOR: A FAMILY INTERVENTION APPROACH

Keith M. Davis, Ph.D., NCC, is a North Carolina Licensed School Counselor and associate professor in the Department of Human Development and Psychological Counseling, Appalachian State University, Boone, NC. Prior to his work as a counselor educator, he was a school counselor. His research interests are professional school counselors providing time-limited family counseling in the schools, male development over the lifespan, and incorporating nature and the outdoors into counseling practice.

CHAPTER 8: SUICIDE ISSUES

Jill Packman, PhD., RPT-S, NCC has been a professor of Counseling at UNR since July 2002. Dr. Packman, associate professor, came to Reno from Texas where her major areas of interest were school counseling and play therapy. Dr. Packman has worked continuously in schools since 1995 both as a counselor and teacher. Since arriving at UNR, Dr. Packman has been recognized for her research by the American Counseling Association and the Association for Play Therapy. She has also been honored by the College of Education as an Outstanding Mentor and by the university being awarded one of the first Silver Compass Awards.

Ms. Catey Barber is a professional school counselor at O'Brien Middle School, Reno, NV. She has worked in schools since 1999 and has been a school counselor since 2004. Ms. Barber was always drawn to "at-risk" students choosing to work and help students in challenging settings. This passion has motivated her to take a special interest in researching issues that she encounters on a daily basis.

CHAPTER 9: LEARNING DISABILITIES

Glenn W. Lambie, Ph.D., LPC, NCC, NCSC, CCMHC, is an associate professor and school counseling coordinator in the Counselor Education Program at the University of Central Florida. He earned his Master's degree in Counselor Education from Virginia Commonwealth University, an advanced certificate in Professional Counseling from the Medical College of Virginia/VCU, and a doctoral degree in Counselor Education from The College of William & Mary. Dr. Lambie has worked in the counseling profession for 15 years as a counselor educator, professional school counselor, and family and individual therapist. He has published significantly in the areas of professional school counseling, counselor development and supervision, and counseling children and adolescent "at-risk" populations. Dr. Lambie has served on the ASCA Ethics Committee and on the editorial boards of *Professional School Counseling* (ASCA) and the *Journal of Counseling and Development* (ACA).

Kara P. Ieva, M.Ed, NCC, NCSC, is a doctoral candidate in the Counselor Education Program at the University of Central Florida. She earned her Master's degree in school counseling from Loyola College in Baltimore, Maryland. Ms. Ieva has worked for 10 years in education both as a Spanish teacher and as a professional school counselor. Ms Ieva currently works as a professional school counselor at both the middle school and high school levels, providing individual and group counseling and facilitating the delivery of a comprehensive developmental guidance curriculum to a diverse student population. Ms. Ieva's research interests include professional school counseling, urban education, and counseling children and adolescents "at-risk" populations.

Stacy M. Van Horn, Ph.D., is a faculty member in the Counselor Education Program at the University of Central Florida. She earned her doctoral degree in Counselor Education from the University of Florida, Gainesville. Dr. Van Horn has worked in the counseling profession for 12 years as a counselor educator and professional school counselor in the state of Florida. Her primary research interest is professional school counselor preparation and development.

Jonathan H. Ohrt, M.A., is a doctoral candidate in the Counselor Education Program at the University of Central Florida. He earned his Master's degree in Counselor Education at the University of South Florida and worked as a professional school counselor in secondary schools. Mr. Ohrt has published in the *Professional School Counseling* (ASCA) journal and his research foci include counselor development, group counseling, and school counselor effectiveness.

Sally V. Lewis, M.Ed., NCC, NCSC, is a doctoral candidate in the Counselor Education Program at the University of Central Florida. She earned her Master's degree in Education in Secondary Guidance with coursework in Elementary Counseling from the University of South Carolina. Ms. Lewis has worked in the professional school counseling profession for over 13 years as a professional school counselor at the elementary school level. Prior to working as a school counselor, Ms. Lewis was an exceptional education teacher and staffing specialist. Her areas of research include professional school counseling and counseling children and adolescents, particularly those with special needs.

B. Grant Hayes, Ph.D., LPC, NCC, is a professor of counselor education and the associate dean for Graduate Studies in the College of Education at the University of Central Florida. He earned his Master's degree in school counseling, and an Educational Specialist (Ed.S.) degree in counselor education and a Ph.D. in Counselor Education and Supervision from the University of South Carolina at Columbia. Dr. Hayes has worked in the counseling profession for 20 years as a counselor educator and professional school counselor. He is a past-president of the Counseling Association for Humanistic Education and Development (C-AHEAD) and serves as a board member for the Association for Spiritual, Ethical, and Religious Values in Counseling (ASERVIC). Additionally, Dr. Hayes serves on the ACA Advisory Editorial Board and the editorial boards of *Counselor Education and Supervision* (ACES) and the *Journal for Counseling and Development* (ACA).

Index

Note: Page numbers in *Italic* indicate tables.

A

Absenteeism, *96*
Academy of Eating Disorders, 67, *81*
Accommodations, *160*
Acting-out behaviors, 123–133
  case study, 124
  characteristics, 125
  diagnostic features, 125
  influencing factors, 125
  overview, 123–124, 133
  prevalence, 125
  resources, 131–133
  See also Interventions
ACTION, 27–*28*
Action stage, 99
Adderall, 9
ADD–H Comprehensive Teacher's
  Rating Scale (ACTeRS), 8
ADD Warehouse, *13*
Adequate Yearly Progress (AYP), 3, *160*
Adolescent Suicide Interview, 144
Aggressive behaviors
  assessment, 23
  case study, 17
  as disorder, 18
  factors influencing, 18
  identification, 18
  mapping, 19
  overview, 16–17
  peers and, 27
  prior history toward, 22
  psychological context for, 23
  strategies for improvement, 29
  See also Violent tendencies
Al-Anon, *101*
Alateen, *101*
Alcoholics Anonymous, *101*
Alliance for Eating Disorder Awareness
  (The Alliance), *81*
Ambivalence, 100
American Academy of Child & Adolescent
  Psychiatry, *55*
American Academy of Pediatrics
  (AAP), 107
American Association for Marriage and
  Family Therapy, *55*
American Association for Suicidology, *149*
American Foundation for Suicide
  Prevention, *149*
American Psychiatric Association (APA),
  2, 39, 18, 139
American School Counselor Association
  (ASCA), 23, 50, 132, 167, *168*
American Self-Harm Clearinghouse, *55*
Americans with Disabilities Act (ADA)
  of 1990
  and body image relationship, *68*

and eating disorder relationship, *68*
learning disablities, 159
overview, *160*, 162
Anorexia Nervosa (AN), 66
Anorexia Nervosa and Related Eating
    Disorders, *81*
Anxiety
    case study, 37
    disorders, 39–40
    mental health screening plan, 46–47
    onset age, 40–43
    overview, 36–38, 54
    peer support, 48
    personal fears and, 44
    Positive Behavior Support (PBS), 45–46
    prevalence rates, 40, 44
    prevention, 47–50
    referral and supportive counseling, 49
    resources for, *55–56*
    school difficulties, fears and, 44
    school nurse and medication issues,
        49–*50*
    short-term adjustment issues, 44
    small group counseling, 48
    special educational language, 44
    systemic-ecological prevention tools,
        47–48
    warning signs, 39
    See also Interventions; School
        counseling practices
Anxiety disorders (OCD), *43*
Appearance, unkempt, *96*
Argumentation, avoidance, 100
Assessment
    of behaviors, 20–27
    comprehensive behavioral, *24–25*
    instruments for, 21
    liability reduction, 21
    multi-disciplinary teams, 21
    process, 21–27
    risk, 21–23, 27
    suicide risk, 143–146
Assessment instruments for externalizing
    behaviors in school-age children and
    youth, *24–25*
Attention Deficit Disorders Association
    (ADDA), *13*
Attention Deficit Hyperactivity Disorder
    (ADHD) students
    accommodation strategies, 6–7

anticipation of needs of, 7–8
behavioral concerns in, 2
as behavioral disorder, 18
behavior externalization, 18
characteristics, 1
combined, 3
descriptors, *166*
"doing what they know", 5
high school students with, 11–12
identification, 9, 12–13
improvement of academic
    performance, 11
inconsistent performance of, 5
male/female occurrences, 19
overview, 12
predominantly hyperactive-impulsive, 3
    predominantly inattentive, 2
resources for, *13*
school-based case study, 2, 3–4
subtypes, 1–3
types, 2–3
and/or underachievement in, 2
See also Interventions; School counsel-
    ing practices; School psychologists
    and medical professionals
Attitudes that Support or Facilitate
    Violence, *27–28*
Autism, *163*

B

Barber, C., 135
Bardick, A. D., 16, 63
Barkley, Russell, 3
Beck Depression Inventory Second
    Edition (BDI–II), 23, 24
Beck Hopelessness Scale (BHS), 23, *24*
Behavioral disorders (BD), 16–31, 35–56
    assessment, 20–27
    attention-deficit, 18
    case study, 17
    characteristics, 18–19
    classification, 19
    Conduct Disorder (CD), 18–19
    disruptive, 18
    etiology, 19
    externalization of, 16–31
    factors influencing, 19
    identification, 19–20
    internalization of, 35–56

Behavioral disorders (BD) (*continued*)
  interventions, 27–31
  Oppositional Defiant Disorder
    (ODD), 18
  overview, 16, 31
  prevalence, 19
  See also Attention Deficit Hyperactivity
    Disorder (ADHD)
Behavior Assessment System for Children,
  Second Edition (BASC–2), 23, 24
Behavior Intervention Plan (BIP), *160*
Behavior management, 29–30
Bernes, J. I., 16, 63
Bernes, K. B., 16, 63
Binge Eating Disorder (BED), 66
Bipolar II (Hypomanic) disorders, *42*
Body awareness, and acceptance, 68
Body image, 63–81
  assessment, 74
  body awareness, and acceptance, 68
  body paralysis, 69
  body preoccupation, 68–69
  case study, 65
  communicating concerns about, 76–77
  fat-phobic, 73
  improvement strategies, 72–73, 78
  individualized approaches to, 74
  intervention programs, 69–71
  muscle dysmorphia, 66
  overview, 63–65
  participatory approach, 72
  thin ideal and, 70
  topics to address, 71
  unhealthy, 67–69
  See also BRIDGE
Body Image Kits, 71–72
Body-Logic program, 71
Body paralysis, 69
Body piercing, 51
Body preoccupation, 68–69
Body Safety Training, 117
Borderline Personality Disorder (BPD), 51
Bratton, S. C., 171
BRIDGE (Building the Relationship
    between Body Image and Disordered
    Eating Graph and Explanation)
    model, 67–69
Brief family systems approach (BFSA),
    97–98
Brigman, G., 172

Bruce, David S., 116
Bulimia Nervosa (BN), 66
Buspirone (BuSpar), *50*

C

CAGE, 93
Cambron-McCabe, N. H., 170
CANDO, content information memory
    practice, 11
Can't Scream, Can't Shout, *56*
Capacity, 27–*28*
CAPT Team, 147–148
Caregiver concerns, and substance abuse, *96*
Center for Disease Control (CDC), 2
Center for Disease Control and
    Prevention, 137
Center for Mental Health in Schools
    (UCLA), 119
Center for Substance Abuse Prevention, *101*
Centers for Disease Control and
    Prevention (CDC), *13*
Central Auditory Processing Disorder, *166*
Chief enabler, *95*
Child Assault Prevention (CAP), 117
Child Behavior Checklist for Ages 6–18
    (CBCL/6-18), *24*
Child Maltreatment 2004 report, 109
Child Protective Services (CPS), 107, 108
Children and Adults with ADHD
    (CHADD), *13*
Children of alcoholics, 93–94
  brief family systems approach
    (BFSA), 97–98
  consequences, 93–94
  familial education, 98
  family roles, *95*
  overview, 93
  process versus content, 98
  school-based indicators of, *96*
  systemic liaison, 98
  warning signs, 94
Child sexual abuse. *See* Sexual abuse
Child Study Team, *160*
Child Suicide Potential Scale, 144
"chunking" assignments, 4
Circularity construct, 97
Clinical- versus school-based
    interventions, 146–147
Clomipramine (Anafranil), *50*

Clonazepam (Klonopin), *50*
Clonidine (Catapres), *50*
Cognitive-Behavioral Therapy (CBT),
    49, 80
Cognitive-socio-emotional skills, 447
Collaborative consultations, 126–127
    combined type, 2
    learning disabilities and, 168, 170
Complementarity construct, 97
Comprehensive evaluation, *167*
Comprehensive list of child and adolescent
    appropriate screening instruments, *149*
Comprehensive school counseling
    program (CSCP), 44
Conduct Disorder (CD), 18
Conduct Problems Prevention Group, 18
Conduct Problems Prevention Research
    Group, 18
Conner's Rating Scale Revised
    (CRS-R), 8
Contemplation stage, 99–100
Cornell decision-tree model, 22
Cornell University, 51
Council for Exceptional Children (CEC),
    13, 156, *168*, 172
Crescent Life, Self Injury, *56*
Cyclothymic disorders, *42*

D

Davis, K. M., 123–133
Deaf-blindness (DB), *163*
Deafness, *163*
Deliberate self-harming (DSH), 51
Dennison, J., 11
Depression
    case study, 37
    characteristics, 38–38
    disorders, 39–40
    mental health screening plan, 46–47
    onset age, 40–43
    overview, 36–38, 54
    peer support, 48
    Positive Behavior Support (PBS), 45–46
    prevalence rates, 40, 44
    prevention, 47–50
    referral and supportive counseling, 49
    resources for, *55–56*
    school nurse and medication issues, 49–*50*
    small group counseling, 48

special educational language, 44
symptoms, *50*
warning signs, 38–39
Depressive disorders, *41*
Developmental Pathways Screening
    Program (DPSP), 93
Dexedrine, 9
*Diagnostic and Statistical Manual of Mental
    Disorders, Text Revision*
    (DSM–IV–TR) 2, 18, 39–43, 67,
    125, 139
Dieting, 75
Disciplinary problems, *96*
Discrepancies, perceiving, 100
Disruptive behavior. *See* Acting-out
    behaviors
Doe v. Rains Independent School
    District, 115
Dr. Barkley, *13*
Dr. Goldstein, *13*
Drug Resistance Abuse Education, *101*
Dyscalculia, *166*
Dysgraphia, *166*
Dyslexia, *166*
Dyspraxia, *166*

E

Earley, B., 172
Early Assessment Risk List for Boys
    (EARL-20B), *25*
Early Assessment Risk List for Girls
    (EARL-21G), *25*
Eating disorders, 63–81
    assessment, 74–76
    case study, 65
    characteristics, 65–69
    communicating with at-risk students
        and caregivers, 76–79
    identification, 74
    long-term outcomes, 66
    medical focus, 78
    overview, 63–65
    prevalence, 66
    prevention, 69–73
    psychological focus, 78–79
    recovery, 69
    relapse prevention, 79
    resource websites, *81*
    self-injurious behavior (SIB) and, 51

Eating disorders (*continued*)
  subtypes, 66
  warning signs, 75
Educational planning, 30–31
Education of All Handicapped Children
    Act of 1975, 159, 162
Ellis, E., 11
Emotional and behavioral disorder (EBD),
    19, 44
Emotional Disturbance (ED), 40, 44, *163*
Empathy, 100
Ethical issues
  case study, 114
  learning disabilities and, 172
  medication issues, 49
  notification of Self-Injurious Behavior
    (SIB) cases, 53
  professional competencies
    and, 53
  sexual abuse, 107, 112–115
  suicidal individuals and, 146
Etiology, 19
Evidence-based practice with
    emotionally troubled children
    and adolescents, 55
Exceptional education legislation,
    162–165
Exceptional education terms, acronyms,
    and definitions, *160–161*
Extended School Year Services
    (ESY), *160*

F

Facilitating systemic change construct, 97
Familial education, and substance abuse, 98
Family Center for Technology and
    Disabilities, 156, *168*
Family hero, *95*
Family history, 21–22
Family interventions. *See* Interventions
Family mascot, *95*
Family Resource Center on
    Disabilities, *168*
Family scapegoat, *95*
Fasting, 75
First Step to Success and Parent-Teacher
    Action Research (PTAR), 46–47
504 plan, 44
Fluoxetine (Prozac), *50*

Fluvoxamine (Luvox), *50*
Food
  allergies, 75
  obsessive rumination, 75
  refusing, 75
Forgan, J. W., 169
Free Appropriate Public Education
    (FAPE), 162, *160*
Functional Behavior Assessment (FBA), *160*

G

Generalized Anxiety Disorder, 22
Goldstein, Sam, 12
Good faith reporting, 113
Good Touch/Bad Touch, 117
Greenberg, K. R., 172
Group interventions, *167*
Guided imagery, 80

H

Handbook of depression in children and
    adolescents, 55
Handicap discrimination, 159
Harley, M. T., 169
Hayes, G., 154
Healthy-Schools, Healthy Kids, 71
Healthy Weight Network, *81*
Hearing Impairment (HI), *163*
*Helping students overcome depression and
    anxiety: A practical guide*, 55
Homeostasis construct, 97
Horowitz, S. H., 169–170
Hypoglycaemia, 75

I

Ieva, K. P., 154
*If your adolescent has an anxiety disorder:
    An essential resource for parents*, 55
*If your adolescent has depression or bipolar
    disorder: An essential resource for
    parents*, 55
Imaginative-constructivist model,
    127–128
Impulse control, poor, *96*
Inclusion (Mainstreaming), *160*
Independent Education Evaluation,
    (IEEF), *160*

Individual Education Plans,
    (IEPs), 7–8
Individualized Education Program
    (IEP), *161*
Individuals with Disabilities Act (IDEA),
    44, 45
Individuals with Disabilities Education
    Improvement Act (IDEIA), 159,
    160–167
  defined, *160*
  diagnoses, 165–167
  disability conditions, *163–164*
  federal legislation, 162
  legal issues, 159
  Response to Intervention (RTI),
    165–167
  specific disabilities, *166*
  transition services, *161*
  triennial reevaluation, *161*
Information Processing Disorder, *166*
Input processing, 156
Integration or organization
    processing, 156
Intelligence Scale for Children, 165
Intensive interventions, *167*
Intent, 27–*28*
International Association of Marriage and
    Family Counselors (IAMFC), 132
International Consensus Statement on
    Attention Deficit Hyperactivity
    Disorder (ADHD), 5
International Dyslexia Association, *168*
Interventions, 7, 9–12, 47–48, 53–54, 77,
    78–81, 116–119, 126–131, 146–148,
    167–170
  acting out behaviors, 126–131
  anxiety and depression, 47–48
  behavior disorders, 27–31
  child sexual abuse, 116–119
  clinical- versus school based, 146–147
  collaboration, 53–54
  consultations, 53
  eating disorders, 79–81
  example of, 10
  family, 126–131
  follow-up meetings, 54
  goals, 48
  high school students with Attention
    Deficit Hyperactivity Disorder
    (ADHD), 11–12

  individual supportive counseling, 54
  medical focus, 78
  notifications, 53
  phases, 78–79
  planning interventions for Attention
    Deficit Hyperactivity Disorder
    (ADHD), 7, 9–12
  postvention, 147–148
  psychological focus, 78–79
  recovery support, 77–78
  referrals, 49, 53, 77
  relapse prevention, 79
  resources, *13, 168*
  Response to Intervention (RTI),
    48, 165–167
  by school counselors, 9–12
  Self-Injurious Behavior (SIB), 53–54
  self-monitoring strategies, 11
  Stop and Think program, 12
  suicide, 146–147
  supportive, 49
  systemic collaborative consultants,
    168–170
  See also specific types
Interviews, 21, 22–23
  Adolescent Suicide Interview, 144
  Child Suicide Potential Scale, 144
  family, 127
  initial, 110
  motivational, 98–*101*
  multiple informants, 21
  overview, 22–23
  scripted, 144
  sexual abuse, 108, 111–112
  structured, 74, 76
  Suicidal Behavioral Inventory, 144
  suicide, 144–145
  third parties during, 116
  violent tendencies, 23

J

Joining, as supporting family
    relationships, 97
Journal for Specialists in Group Work, 48

K

Kampwirth, T. J., 169
Keeping kids safe, healthy, and smart, 55

Kendall, Philip, 12
Kid & Teen SAFE, 118–119
Kidder, K. R., 9

L

Lair, G. S., 171
Lambie, G. W., 87–102, 154, 171
Language Learning Disability (LLD), *161*
LDOnline (Web site on learning
    disabilities), *168*
Learning disabilities (LD), 154–167
    case study, 15
    characteristics, 156–158
    defining, 156
    legal issues, 159–167
    overview, 154
    prevalence, 156–157
    processing dysfunctions, 156
    prognosis, 157
    warning signs, 157–158
Learning Disabilities Association of
    America (LDA), 156, *168*, 172
Least Restrictive Environment (LRE), *161*
Legal issues
    learning disabilities, legislation, 159
    mandated reporters, 113
    sexual abuse, 112–113
    state statutes, 113
Lenz, B., 11
Lesesne, C. A., 2
Let's Talk About Touching, 117
Lewis, S., 154
Lexington Center for the Deaf, 119
LifeSigns, *56*
Lost child, *95*
Lysamena Project (religious-based
    information), *55*

M

Maintenance stage, 99
Manifestation Determination, *161*
Mapping, 19
Mayo Clinic, *55*
McEachern, A. G., 171
Meals, skipping, *75*
Medical history, 21–22
Medical-induced disorders, *42*
Medications

antidepressants, 138
anxiety disorders, *43*
depression, 147
Dr. Goldstein website, *13*
mood disorders and, *42*
psychopharmacology intervention, 146
psychotropic, *50*
school nurses, 49–50
side effects, 49–50
for suicidal usage, 138, 145
use and monitoring, 4, 9, 29, *50*
Memory, 156
Mental Health Association of America,
    13, *55*
Mental Retardation (MR), *163*
Men Who Self-Injure, *56*
Merrill, K. M., 19
Methylphenidate, 9
Miller, W., 171
Millon Adolescent Clinical Inventory
    (MACI), 23, *25*
Milsom, A., 169, 171
Mood disorders, 41–*43*, 139
Motivational counseling (MC), 98–100
Motivational Enhancement
    Therapy, 98
Motivational Interviewing, 98, *101*
Motivational principles, 100
Multi-disciplinary team, 21
Multiple Disabilities (MD), *163*
Muscle dysmorphia, 66
Myers, H. N., 168
Myrick, R. D., 10

N

Nadeau, K., 12
Narrative therapy, 80–81
National Association for Anorexia Nervosa
    and Associated Eating Disorders, *81*
National Association for Children of
    Alcoholics, *101*
National Center for Learning Disabilities
    (NCLD), 165, *168*, 172
National Center for PTSD, *56*
National Center for Special Education
    Personnel and Related Service
    Providers, *168*
National Child Abuse and Neglect Data
    System (NCANDS), 109

National Council on Alcoholism and Drug Dependence, 191
National Dissemination Center for Children with Disabilities (NICHCY), 44, 156, 157, 165
National Eating Disorder Information Center, *81*
National Eating Disorders Association (NEDA), 71, *81*
National Information Center for Children and Youth with Disabilities, *13, 168*
National Institute of Mental Health (NIMH), *13*, 36, *55*, *81*, *149*
National Institute on Alcohol Abuse and Alcoholism, *101*
National Institute on Drug Abuse, *101*
National Model (ASCA, 2005), 171
National Research Center on Learning Disabilities, 157
National Resource Center on AD/HD (NRC): A Program of CHADD (Children and Adults with Attention-Deficit/Hyperactivity Disorder), *13*
National Student Assistance Association, *101*
National Survey on Drug Use and Health (NSDUH), 90
Nefazodone (Serzone), *50*
No Child Left Behind Act, 3
No-Go-Tell Protection Curriculum for Young Children, 119
Non-Compliance with Risk Reduction Interventions category, *27–28*
Nonsuicidal (NSSI) causes, 51–52

O

Obesity, 63–81
    beliefs about, 70, 72
    case study, 65
    overview, 63–65
    prevention program, 71
    See also Body image
Observations, of student behavior, 20
Obsessive-compulsive disorders (OCD), *43*
Office of Special Education Programs (OSEP), *161*
Ohrt, J. H., 154
Oppositional Defiant Disorder (ODD), 18
Orthopedic Impairment (OI), *163*

Other Health Impairment (OHI), *164*
Other's Reactions and Responses, *27–28*
Our Children's Future, 119
Output processing, 156
Oxford handbook of anxiety and related disorders, 55

P

Packman, J., 135, 171
Pain disorders, *42–43*
Parent in-services, depression training, 47
Parents of Attention Deficit Hyperactivity Disorder (ADHD) children
    child management, 7
    concerns of, 3–4
    medical consultations, 8–9
    medications, 4
    training for, 5
    working with school counselors, 4
    working with teachers, 2
    workshops, 6
Paroxetine (Paxil), *50*
Pastor, R., 170
Peer cues, and substance abuse, *96*
Performance, inconsistent, *96*
Perou, R., 2
Phobia disorders, *42–43*
Physical symptoms, and substance abuse, 96
Physician's Desk Reference, 49
Planet Health, 71
Positive Behavior Support (PBS), 45–46
Post Traumatic Stress Disorder, 22
Posttraumatic Stress disorders (PTSD), *43*
Precontemplation stage, 99–100
    predominantly hyperactive-impulsive type, 3
    predominantly inattentive type, 2
Prevalence, 19
Preventing Sexual Abuse: Activities and Strategies for Those Working with Children and Adolescents, 118
Prevention
    Child Abuse and Neglect Prevention, 112
    eating disorders, 69–73
    mental health screening and, 46–47
    parent/caregiver education as, 98
    prevention programs, ineffectual, 142
    Prevention Researcher, *56*

Prevention (*continued*)
  relapse prevention and, 78, 79
  school counselors and, 63, 81
  school-based, 45, 52–53, 54
  sexual abuse, 116–119
  strategies, 47–50
  substance abuse, 94, 101
  suicide, 52, 138, 141–143
  See also specific types
Private Parts, 117
Process, versus content, 98
Professional School Counselor and Child
  Abuse and Neglect Prevention
  position statement (ASCA), 112
Propranolol (Inderal), *50*

Q

QPR Institute, 143

R

Ray, K. E., 168
Reactive Attachment Disorder, 22
Red Flag, Green Flag People, 117–118
Reddy, L. A., 46, 47
Rehabilitation Act, Section 504, 44, 159
Resistance, 100
Remember, 117
Research Program on Self-Injurious
  Behavior in Adolescents and Young
  Adults, 51
Resources
  acting-out behaviors, resources,
    131–133
  for anxiety, *55–56*
  for Attention Deficit Hyperactivity
    Disorder (ADHD) students, *13*
  Center for Mental Health in
    Schools, 119
  Center for Substance Abuse
    Prevention, 94
  for depression, *55–56*
  eating disorders, *81*
  elementary school screening
    programs, 46
  Gateway to a World of Resources for
    Enhancing Mental Health, 119
  intervention programs, 46
  for learning disabilities, *168*

Motivational Counseling (MC)
  therapeutic strategies, 100
National Resource Center on
  AD/HD (NRC): A Program
  of CHADD (Children and Adults
  with Attention-Deficit/Hyperactivity
  Disorder), *13*
Parent Teacher Association, 143
Professional school counselors, web
  sites, *149*
School-based Violence Prevention
  Programs: A Resource Manual, 117
for school counseling, *55–56*
school psychologist as, 8
for self-injurious behavior (SIB), *55–56*
substance abuse, *101*
for suicide, 149
Suicide Prevention Basics, 142
Student Assistance Team Manual, 46
Respect, 100
Response to Intervention (RTI), *161*,
  165–167
Richardson, L., 46, 47
Right Health.com, *56*
Risk assessment, 26–27
Ritalin (methylphenidate), 9
Rogers, C. R., 171
Russell-Mayhew, S., 63

S

S.A.F.E. Alternatives, *56*
Sad affect, *96*
Safe Child, 118
SAMHSA's National Clearinghouse for
  Alcohol & Drug Information, *101*
Schechtman, Z., 170
School-based Violence Prevention
  Programs: A Resource Manual, 117
School counseling practices, 4–8, 45–50,
  69–76
  accommodation of needs for Attention
    Deficit Hyperactivity Disorder
    (ADHD), 7
  acknowledgement of Attention Deficit
    Hyperactivity Disorder (ADHD), 5
  acting-out behaviors, resources, 131–133
  anticipation of needs of Attention
    Deficit Hyperactivity Disorder
    (ADHD) students, 7–8

anxiety and depression, 45–50
awareness of the nature and symptoms
    of ADHD, 6–7
eating disorders, 69–76
group counseling, 171–172
learning disabilities, 167–172
as liaisons, 53
as mandatory child abuse
    reporters, 113
manuals for, *24–25*
overview, 12
planning interventions for Attention
    Deficit Hyperactivity Disorder
    (ADHD), 7, 9–12
as a point person, 53
recommendations, 4–8
resources, *55–56, 168*
Response to Intervention (RTI), *167*
services, 170–171
session topics and key points, 10
sexual abuse, 114–119
substance abuse, 94–100
suicide warning signs and, 141–148
as support services coordinator, 53
See also Interventions
School history, 22
School nurses, 49–50
School psychologists and medical
    professionals, 8–9
Schwab Foundation, *13*
Schwiebert, V., 11
Screening process, *167*
Sealander, K., 11
Secret Shame, *56*
Section 504 of the Rehabilitation Act
    of 1973, 159, *161*
Section 504. *See* 504 plan
Self-efficacy, 100
Self-injurious behavior (SIB), 50–54
    case study, 50
    characteristics, 51
    correlates, 51–52
    nonsuicidal (NSSI) causes, 51–52
    overview, 50–51, 52, 54
    prevalence rates, 51
    prevention, 52–53
    resources for, *55–56*
    suicidal (SSI) and, 53
    See also Interventions
Self-Injury and Related Issues, *56*

Self-Injury: A Struggle, 56
Self-Injury Information and Support, *56*
Self-monitoring strategies, 11
Sertraline (Zoloft), *50*
Sexual abuse, 106–119
    assessment, 107–108
    case study, 106, 114
    developmentally normal behavior,
        107–109
    ethical issues, 112, 114–115
    incident level, 109
    interviews, 111–112
    legal, 112–113
    overview, 106–107, 119
    prevention, 116–119
    in schools, 115–116
    state statutes, 113
    student disclosure, 110–111
    warning signs, 109–112
    See also Interventions
Sexual development, 107–108
Sexual identity, 141
Sexual offenders, tactics of, 116
Shillingford, M. A., 9
Sias, 90
Sink, C. A., 35–56
Smith, I. C., 171
Socio-economic status (SES), 40
Specific Learning Disability (SLD or LD),
    161, 164
Speech or Language Impairment (SI), *164*
Sridhar, D., 169
Standardized assessment instruments,
    23–26
States for Treatment Access and Research
    (STAR) program, 71
Stimulants, 9
Stop and Think program, 12
Stone, C., 106–119
Straterra, 9
Stress, 140–141
    Acute Stress Disorder, *43*
    binging and, 80
    guided imagery technique, 80
    improvement, 29
    interviewing for, 22
    management, 30, 47, 49, 53, 69, 71, 72
    overview, 140–141
    Post Traumatic Stress Disorder (PSTD),
        22, 36, 40, *43, 50*

Stress (*continued*)
  prevention programs, ineffectual, 142
  recovery stage and, 54
  relapse prevention and, 79
  suicidal ideation and, 139
  triggers, 79
Structural-strategic family counseling,
    128–131
  family reorganization, 129
  goals, 128
  overview, 128
  parents, working with, 129–131
  time-limited, 128
Structured Assessment of Violence and
    Risk in Youth (SAVRY), 23, *25*, 26
Structured Judgment Approach, 21
Structured Professional Judgment, 26
Student behavioral reports, 20
Student collaboration
  at-risk for Self-Injurious Behavior (SIB),
    52–54
  behavior management, 29–30
  developmental competencies, 47
  eating disorders, 76–77
  educational/vocational planning, 30–31
    emotional disturbance (ED), 44
  medication issues, 49–50
  observations of, 20, 39
  peer support, 48
  prosocial skill strategies, 45–46
  sexual abuse disclosures, 110–111
  Student Assistance Team Manual, 46
  support systems for, 45
  See also Attention Deficit Hyperactivity
    Disorder (ADHD) students;
    Interventions
Study buddies, 4
Substance abuse, 87–102
  case study, 88–89
  characteristics, 89–90
  consequences, 91
  educational indicators, *92*
  familial characteristics, *92*
  identification, 91–93
  overview, 87–89, 101–102
  prevalence, 90
  psychological cues, *92*
  resources, *101*
  and suicide, 140
  warning signs, 89–90, 91–93

Substance Abuse and Mental Health
    Services Administration (SAMHSA),
    90, 94, *101*
Substance Abuse Subtle Screening
    Inventory—Adolescent 2
    (SASSI—A2), 93
Substance-induced disorders, *42–43*
Suicidal (SSI), 51
Suicidal Behavioral Inventory, 144
Suicidal Ideation Questionnaire
    (SIQ), 144
Suicide, 135–149
  attempted, 137
  background information, 137–141
  case study, 136
  characteristics, 138–141
  EndingSuicide.com, 144
  family influences, 139–140
  ideations, *24*, 137, 145
  measures, 23, *25*
  mood disorders, 139
  overview, 136–137, 148
  prevalence, 137–138
  prevention, 141–143
  resources, 149
  risk assessment, 143–146
  sexual identity, 141
  social relationships, 139–140
  stress, 140–141
  substance abuse, 140
  Suicide Probability Scale
    (SPS), *25*
  threatened, 137
  warning signs, 138–141
  See also Interventions
Suicide Prevention Basics, 142
Suicide Prevention Resource Center,
    142, *149*
Suicide Probability Scale, (SPS),
    23, *25*, 144
Supportive Self-Help Web Sites, *56*
Surgeon General mental health
    report, 40
Surprises, 117
Systematic Screening for Behavior
    Disorders process (SSBD), 46
Systemic consultations, 126–127,
    168–170
Systemic interventions, *167*
Systemic liaison, 98

T

Tardiness, *96*
Targeted interventions, *167*
Taylor, C., 171
Teachers
  awareness of the nature and symptoms
    of Attention Deficit Hyperactivity
    Disorder (ADHD), 6–7
  behavioral reports, 20
  helping to acknowledge Attention
    Deficit Hyperactivity Disorder
    (ADHD), 5
  identification of externalizing
    behaviors, 19
  in-services, 143
  learning disabilities and, 158
  Parent-Teacher Action Research
    (PTAR), 46
  Parent-Teacher association, 143
  -parent workshops, for Attention
    Deficit Hyperactivity Disorder
    (ADHD) students, 6
  rating scales, 8
  reports, 20
  social difficulties, 4
  underachievement, 3
  See also School counseling practices
TEAM, 147–148
Tell Someone, 117
The Capital, 115–116
The Family Journal, 132
*The Prevention Researcher, By Parents for
    Parents*, 56
Therapies
  art, 30, 171
  bibliotherapy, 169
  Cognitive-Behavioral Therapy
    (CBT), 80
  Guided imagery, 80
  Motivational counseling (MC), 98–100
  Narrative therapy, 30, 80–81
  outpatient, 54
  play, 30, 171
  talk, 30
  Transtheoretical Model of Change
    (TMC), 99–100
  See also specific types
Thresholds Crossed, 27–28
Transition Services, *161*

Transtheoretical Model of Change
    (TMC), 99–100
Traumatic Brain Injury (TBI), *164*
Treating child and adolescent
    depression, 55
Treating self-injury: A practical guide, 55
Triennial Reevaluation, *161*

U

U.S. Department of Education Office for
    Civil Rights, 4
U.S. Department of Health and Human
    Services, *101*
U.S. Department of Special Education
    Practice, 8
U.S. Office of Special Education Practice, *13*
Ungame Teen Card Game, 171
Unkempt appearance, *96*

V

Van Horn, S., 154
Vaughn, S., 169
Vegetarian diet, *75*
Very Important Kids, 71
Violent tendencies
  ACTION, *28*
  case study, 17
  differentiation from normal behavior, 18
  domestic, 18, 22
  factors influencing, 18
  interviews, 23
  mapping, 19
  overview, 16–17, 31
  risk assessment, 21–23, 27, *28*
  support for, 27
  See also Aggressive behaviors
Visser, S. N., 2
Visual Impairment including Blindness
    (VI), *164*
Visual Processing Disorder, *166*
Vocational planning, 30–31
Volker, T., 168

W

Warning signs
  for anxiety, 39

Warning signs (*continued*)
for children of alcoholics, 94
for depression, 38–39
for eating disorders, *75*
for learning disabilities, 157–158
for sexual abuse, 109–112
for substance abuse, 89–90, 91–93
for suicide, 138–141

Webb, L. D., 1–13
Wegscheider-Cruse, 94
West, J., 171
Williams, W. C., 171

Z

Zentall, S., 6